Introduction to the Anatomy and Physiology of Children

Janet MacGregor

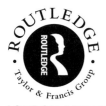

ROUTLEDGE

LONDON AND NEW YORK

First published 2000
by Routledge
11 New Fetter Lane, London EC4P 4EE

Simultaneously published in the USA and
Canada
by Routledge
29 West 35th Street, New York, NY 10001

Reprinted 2001

*Routledge is an imprint of the Taylor & Francis
Group*

© 2000 Janet MacGregor

Typeset in Janson and Futura by Routledge
Printed and bound in Great Britain by
St Edmundsbury Press, Bury St Edmunds,
Suffolk

British Library Cataloguing in Publication Data
A catalogue record for this book is available
from the British Library

*Library of Congress Cataloging-in-Publication
Data*
MacGregor, Janet
Introduction to the anatomy and physiology
of children/Janet MacGregor.
p cm.
Includes bibliographical references and index.
1. Children–Physiology. 2. Human anatomy.
3. Child development. I. Title. [DNLM: 1.
Child Development. 2. Anatomy–Child.
3. Anatomy–Infant. 4. Physiology–Child.
5. Physiology–Infant. WS 103 M146i 2000]
RJ125.M23   2000
612'.0083–dc21   99–34182
DNLM/DLC   CIP

ISBN 0–415–21508–0 (hbk)
ISBN 0–415–21509–9 (pbk)

WS 103

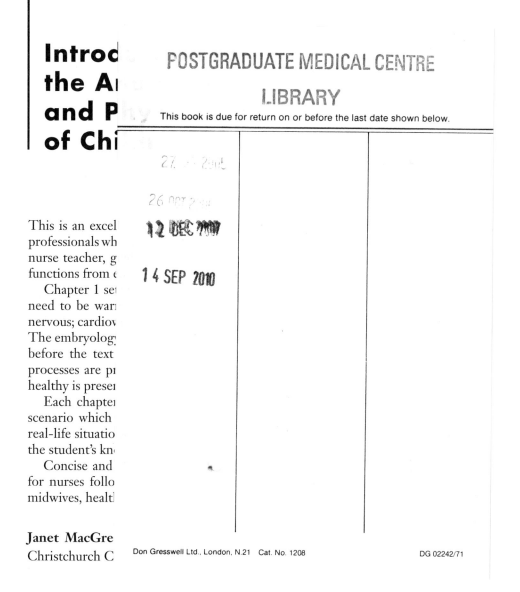

Introd
the A
and P
of Chi

This is an excel
professionals wh
nurse teacher, g
functions from

   Chapter 1 se
need to be war
nervous; cardiov
The embryolog
before the text
processes are p
healthy is prese

   Each chapte
scenario which
real-life situatio
the student's kn

   Concise and
for nurses follo
midwives, healt

Janet MacGre
Christchurch C

15-99

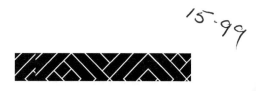

This book is dedicated to my students and the children we care for.

I am particularly grateful to four 'little people', whom I have studied closely in compiling this book:

Morgan
George
Annabel
Hamish

May these reflections on your individual development help those who are interested in other children's physical development to understand all children's needs and thus provide the optimum environment for them to achieve their unique genetic potential.

Thank you.

Contents

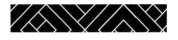

Illustrations

Figures

Tables

Preface

This book is not a comprehensive guide to children's physical development, but an introduction to some selected topics commonly discussed with students working in child health contexts, and for parents who wish to provide the optimum environment for their offspring to flourish.

There is a wide range of 'normal' at any age, no more so than in the period before adult attributes are attained. However, there are physical milestones that all children reach in a definite sequence, and these milestones are universal.

Most parents note the age their baby rolls and sits; most teachers know which skills their pupils should be able to perform; most health professionals know the parameters of their small charges' vital signs.

The content of this book, which is for parents, teachers and health professionals, will first set the scene for physical development to take place. Two development theories have been chosen which present the nature–nurture effect on physical change. Some selected topics are then addressed, such as healthy environments and health promotion issues, which should facilitate children's optimal growth. The succeeding chapters then investigate the body systems in more detail, where it is hoped the reader will be stimulated to take their own interest further and research some of the topics more fully. The final chapter takes the reader back from the physical to the psychological, and thus completes the circle, where a healthy body is intricately entwined with a happy child.

Chapter 1

Child physical needs

- Child development theories
- The nature–nurture debate
- Genetic inheritance
- A healthy environment
- The need for protective care
- Immunisation
- Healthy diet
- Keeping warm
- Exercise

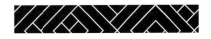

T HE PHYSICAL DEVELOPMENT of children is part of their whole development and therefore must be seen in the context of the social, emotional and intellectual changes that occur through childhood. Child development theories reflect the philosophies of their various authors, but as the subject is so complex, these have often been formulated from a particular stance. For this discussion, two theories have been selected to support the genetic and environmental effects on physical change. Inherited influences can be both subtle and obvious, as can the more long-term effects of environment. The effects of both interact over many years from conception to adult status; they are instrumental in changing the child as it physically grows and matures.

Child development theories

Bee (1997) suggests that there are three fundamental child development concepts that need to be understood:

- the way in which children are the same and different
- the internal and external influences on these changes
- whether changes are quantitative or qualitative in nature

To this end, there are two groups of theories on development that are helpful in understanding the changes that occur in the 'physical' child, and reflect the internal and external nature of the influences for change. These are the biological theories and the learning theories.

Biological theories are based on common patterns of development and the unique individual behavioural tendencies that are partially programmed by genetic inheritance. The development of sitting, for example, occurs as the maturation of systems allows this skill to occur. There is some acknowledgement that the child must be in an environment that facilitates this, and that the child has the inclination to do so.

The biological changes are both quantitative and qualitative in nature; children can be 'aged' by the degree of ossification of their skeletal system. However, their genetic inheritance, the degree of activity they have experienced and their usual diet will ensure children will all be slightly different. It is with this biological philosophy that the succeeding chapters will explore the physical changes that occur in childhood.

The second group of theories comprises the learning theories, which propose that only reflexes are inherited and that all subsequent behaviour changes are learnt. For such theorists, the environmental influence is most important, together with the process within that of learning. The learnt behaviour that takes place can only be inferred from observing the changed behaviour. It is a learnt behaviour that must be relatively permanent and which results from past experience (Gross 1996). These learnt behaviours then become cumulative in nature, and require memory to allow them to develop. They are qualitative in nature – the child can be seen to perform a skill more successfully. Children learning to skip show this qualitative development: at first they cannot coordinate the rope with their feet, but with practice they soon develop sophisticated movements as they work with the rope. A learnt behaviour can also arise from a conditional response, such as the child being praised for eating lunch. This is called the law of effect, where there is a pleasurable experience in performing a task that perhaps is not initiated by the child. Much behaviour therapy uses this technique when the temper tantrum is ignored but the acceptable response rewarded. An alternative learning theory is that of watching rather than doing; the learnt behaviour developing through an interpersonal situation. Here the child will watch a role model and see the consequence of this model's actions. If children value the result of the action they will use the behaviour themselves. Young children watch older children using the toilet and being praised for this action, so they will mimic their behaviour. They also see older children scream and shout to get their own way, and copy this!

The nature–nurture debate

The nature–nurture debate reflects the biological and learning theories discussed above. Inherited and environmental factors are both shown to play an important role in ensuring that the child will develop into a unique individual. Adult height is achieved through the interaction of the inherited potential from both parents, and the child growing in an optimum environment, such as one where they receive adequate nutrition and are free from disease. There have been such environmental changes in most Western populations over the past fifty years, and children at the end of the 1990s are growing taller and maturing earlier. The complex interaction between

3

inheritance and environment may still be seen in changes that occur in recently migrating populations. Those groups who, for example, change their diet and lifestyle, and perhaps marry into the indigenous race when settling into a new country, may see their children's physical growth and maturation change over many future generations (McQuaid *et al.* 1996).

Genetic inheritance

Inherited characteristics are transmitted from one generation to the next in a random way, and they strongly affect the end result of growth and the progress towards it. There is a high correlation with a child and parent regarding height, weight, shape and form of features, body build and skin colour. Many dimensions of personality, such as temperament, also seem to be inherited (Wong 1999). Inherited potential is decided at conception as the genes from both father and mother combine to form the new individual.

Early research established that some genes were dominant to others and held the more likely characteristics to be expressed, such as hair colour and eye colour. Recessive genes, those that were 'hidden' by the dominant genes, provide the 'throwback' phenomenon produced when both parents carry the recessive characteristic. Thus two 'coloured' individuals could produce a black and a white child as siblings. It is now commonly believed that it is not genes that are individually expressed, but the interaction of these inherited characteristics that generally produces many of an individual's features. The unusual colouring of ginger hair and green eyes, or the unexpected stature of a very small son or daughter, may be examples of this phenomenon. Genetically inherited characteristics can also be seen in the distinct racial groups. Afro-Caribbean children develop their muscular skeletal systems in advance of white or Chinese children, regardless of their diet or environment. Black babies hold their heads up well, and may sit and stand earlier than those of other racial groups.

Berger (1998) reports that the Human Genome Project is all set to present the fully sequenced **human genome** in 2003. Apart from the basic sequencing of the genome, and the plan to study human genetic variation and human susceptibility to disease, the Project is also sequencing the genomes of other important organisms, including the mouse, yeast, fruit fly, Japanese puffer fish and roundworm. The collaboration involves Britain, the USA, France, Japan and Germany. New treatments using genetic engineering are already today helping infertile couples to conceive their child using artificially stimulated oogenesis, donated eggs and sperms, and 'wombs for rent'. The cloning of animals has been successful, and the manufacture of medications which replicate the genetic patterning of the natural product is widely practised. Genetic scientists can predict sex and some physical abnormalities: the construction of a human child is not a dream.

A healthy environment

Physical health in children's early years is of paramount importance; they must be given the best possible chance of a healthy future. As they grow and change, so their health needs change for them to achieve their genetic potential. Many factors influence their physical health before and after birth. Children's views about their health also change as they experience the world, adapt and refine their purpose in life. Moules and Ramsey (1998) offer a definition of health taken from developmental psychologists, one which emphasises 'actualisation', the realisation of human potential through purposeful action. They suggest that this developmental approach to health promotion for children is most appropriate, as it parallels the development of cognitive processes. Thus children of six years will see health in a 'concrete' way, as enabling them to do what they want to do: play outside and go to school. The teenager, however, will find the task of defining health more difficult and probe the questioner for context, seeing health as something more 'abstract' that involves both body and mind.

There are projects in cities aimed at making the environment more friendly to children, such as the Healthy Cities Project initiated by the World Health Organisation (WHO). This initiative has now been extended to the worldwide Healthy Cities Movement. One of its targets relates to health-promoting physical and social environments, concentrating professional help into empowering populations to develop skills that allow them to make healthy choices for living (Twinn *et al.* 1998). All children need safe areas for physical play, away from pollution, noise and traffic, and they need to be encouraged to be physically active in activities they enjoy (see Chapters 2–4 on the skeletal, muscular and cardiovascular systems).

The following topics for health promotion are offered as important to optimal physical development:

- the need for protective care
- the need for food
- the need for temperature control
- the need for activity and rest

The need for protective care

Children depend not only on their immediate carers for protection, but on the policies of the state to create a safe environment in which they can thrive. Hall (1996) stressed the importance of promoting child health in the community, and one of his key recommendations was for accident prevention measures. All body systems require freedom from the stresses of pain, anxiety and medical interventions, which are often part of the accident and illness experience, to develop to their full potential. It is when children experience either visible or invisible (biological) harm that the development of their physical self is seen to suffer (see the section on stress in Chapter 9's discussion of the immune system).

Protection from visible risks – accidental and non-accidental injury

Accidental injury

Accidents are the single most reported cause of death in children between the ages of one and fifteen years; children are seen as adventurous, unpredictable and fun-seeking. However, those minor accidents that happen in the home are rarely reported and perhaps are part of growing up. Children can be clumsy, impetuous and curious, and their carers can be ignorant of their needs and lax in supervision. Families may live in poverty and the children be disadvantaged (Fatchcett 1995). Woodroffe *et al.* (1993) however, show that death rates due to all accidents in the UK decreased between 1969 and 1990. They suggest that this may be, in part, due to safer home and local environments, advances in medical science and easy access to health care. However, constant minor injuries and their frequent association with infections that do not kill may result in children expending their energy for tissue repair rather than for growth.

The infant is at risk of falling due to the innate reflexes propelling the child forward, for example, from the baby chair if not strapped in. Babies soon start to roll, and may roll from a changing mat to the floor. At six months, small objects may be ingested or inhaled as the baby grasps and investigates with the mouth. When crawling is achieved, the child will not know that interesting objects on the floor are dangerous to eat.

Young school-aged children are only beginning to understand causal relationships and to think about the effects of their actions. They have improving muscle coordination and want to practise and perfect their physical skills. Cycling is a favourite activity for this age group, but in the excitement of the chase they may forget to watch for cars that share the public domain. They are increasingly exposed to more and various environments, and are easily distracted from a safe course by things that are seen as more interesting.

Teenagers have often progressed to activities involving motorbikes and alcohol, which may frequently lead to involvement in fights. Children of this age group have a need to establish themselves as independent and responsible for their own actions, and this command over their own lives may lead them to feel indestructible. They may not consider the consequences of their actions if peer group pressure is strong. They participate in more sporting activities, and are thus more exposed to physical injury (Wong 1999).

Non-accidental injury

Child abuse is often the result of family stress, a need for parenting skills, and/or children frightened to ask for help. Few single influences on development, however, including severe abuse, have inevitable future consequences for the child. It is the sum and direction of many positive and negative influences that will have a bearing on the eventual outcome of their adjustment in adult life. Physical abuse is the most common single category for 'at risk' registration; the trend is a decline for children under five years and is rising in those aged five to sixteen years. Other categories are sexual, emotional and neglect (Browne 1998; DOH 1991). One of the common indicators of any abuse is that the child will physically fail to thrive (see Chapter 10). Sleep disturbance, eating disorders and 'frozen awareness' are behavioural indicators of children finding difficulty in coping with their lives (Fatchett 1995).

For a child to develop, he or she needs a secure attachment from which to explore the world and to return to when anxious or distressed (Adcock 1998). Fahlberg (1991) gives reasons for the importance of attachment which has an effect as the child 'unfolds' over time in the physical, social and emotional spheres of its life.

The child needs a secure attachment to:

- attain his or her full intellectual potential
- sort out what he or she perceives
- think logically
- develop a conscience
- become self-reliant
- cope with stress and frustration
- handle fear and worry
- develop future relationships
- handle jealousy

Jones (1991) describes a series of key tasks of social and emotional development which interrelate and influence each other:

- the baby's achievement of a balanced physiological state in the first few weeks of life
- the development of a secure attachment with a carer in the first year of life
- the development of an independent sense of self in the first three years of life
- the establishment of peer relationships in the first seven years of life
- the integration of attachment, independence and peer relationships in the first twelve years of life

There appears to be a lack of agreement on the basic nature of childhood among professionals who aim to protect children from harm. The Children Act (1989), in certain circumstances, allows for the child's wishes to be taken into consideration in any action involving them, but the family in which they live may be permitted to have parental responsibility for decision-making, as children are considered to be physically weak, immature and powerless (Harris 1998). This has resulted in professionals needing to control the family in order to protect the child. Child protection is now perceived as distinct from child care, and the product of a relationship between the state, the family and the child to support the child's rights of citizenship.

Protection from invisible (biological) risk

Immunisation

Immunisation programmes are available for all children in the UK. There are nine infections for which protection is routinely offered at present. Today, these diseases are rarely seen; thus parents have become more concerned with the side-effects of the vaccines on healthy children than with the effects of the infections themselves. The debate surrounding the measles, mumps, rubella (MMR) injections suggests, perhaps, that a more enlightened partnership with parents is required by the government of the day. With 25 per cent of children in 1998 (Rejtman 1998) not vaccinated against these infections, it is feared that a major epidemic will occur in three to four years' time, with a whole series of children unnecessarily dying or being damaged in one way or another. Rejtman also suggests that effort in three areas should be made to prevent the crisis from occurring and to address the present anxiety of parents. First, larger and longer-term research must be carried out and the results published to determine if the vaccine or its administration needs to be altered. Second, information which explains the effects of the vaccine, both positive and potentially negative, should be freely available and presented in a clear and concise manner. Third, the government should consider offering the options of separate vaccines so that all children have some protection, rather than, as in the present position, none at all.

The need for food

Dietary habits have shown some healthy trends in the past thirty years. Vegetarianism is on the increase, with 13.3 per cent of sixteen to twenty-four year olds consuming this type of diet (Carter and

Dearmum 1995). There is less red meat, butter, cake and biscuits consumed, and more poultry, fresh fruit and brown bread eaten. A healthy diet should be based on a wide variety of foods, with emphasis on those foods of high nutrient density rather than those providing energy only. This balanced diet can be achieved by selecting items from four food groups each day. Three can be taken from lean meat, fish, poultry, game, eggs, pulses and nuts; three from milk, cheese and yoghurt; four from bread, rice, pasta, breakfast cereal and potatoes; four from vegetables and fruit (National Dairy Council 1995). Chan (1995) describes the Chinese custom of balancing the diet with reference to hot (Yang) and cold (Yin) foods, in order to ensure continuing health and to restore health after illness.

Malnutrition and the subsequent detrimental effect on physical development can result from lack of food, the wrong food and too much food. The effect of diet starts in the womb; the foetus relies on the mother to provide all the necessary nutrients for growth. The baby will grow at the expense of the mother if food is deficient, and Vines (1997) reports that these children, poorly nourished before birth, may later show a reduction of immune function. At birth, the baby can depend on colostrum, a thin, yellowish fluid which is particularly valuable for the establishment of lactobacilli in the gut, and contains less fat and energy but more secretory IgA immunoglobulin than later breast milk. Later mature breast milk, available at ten to fourteen days after birth, is unique in that its composition varies over the course of a feed, a day and the period of lactation. Lactose is the principal carbohydrate of mature breast milk, providing about 39 per cent of the energy for the baby. Proteins composing 60 per cent whey to 40 per cent casein are particularly easily digested, and predominantly long-chain fatty acids provide 50 per cent of all energy requirements until the age of four months, when the gut physiology is matured and weaning to solids can commence. Breast milk also contains a number of anti-infective properties such as macrophages, IgA, lysozyme, lactoferrin, interferon and bifidus factor, which appear to protect the infant from respiratory and gastrointestinal infections in the first few months of life (Rudolf and Leucene 1999). Thompson (1998) suggests that mothers are influenced by friends, knowledge of breast feeding and the way they themselves were fed as babies. The 1990 OPCS survey (White *et al.* 1992) found that the mother's social class, age, education and positive experience of breast feeding were lso important in the choice of breast or bottle. Bottle feeding of infant formula is a safe alternative if all the hygiene and preparation instructions are followed; however, cow's full fat pasteurised milk is not suitable for those infants under one year, as the sodium content is too high and the iron content is too low for their nutritional requirements. The composition of all infant milk formulas in the UK complies with government guidelines of the 1995 regulations (DOH 1995).

Weaning presents an early challenge to both mother and child. Different tastes and textures have to be experienced gradually, in order that the child will accept a varied diet and thus the range of nutrients for optimal growth. Formula milk alone, although continuing as an important source of nourishment for the growing baby, will not provide enough energy for the four to six month old child; by this age their stores of iron and zinc, important for red blood cell function and immune system response, will be low. Lumps in food are needed to stimulate chewing and development of the jaw, which is vital for the later function of speech. Food refusal, faddy feeding and mealtime battles are common at the one to three year stage, but if sweet drinks and crisps are not offered as substitutes for meals, children will eventually accept a range of nutritious foods to keep them healthy as they grow through their early childhood. Some of the more restricted menus, such as baked beans, bread, bananas and fish fingers, are better than canned fizzy drinks and salty snacks.

The nutritional standards requirements for schools was abandoned in 1980 (Carter and Dearmum 1995). This has resulted in widespread development of cafeteria-style school lunches of a snack-type nature, even at five years of age when children enter the education system. Children can be seen to purchase 'tasty' food that is high in fat and sugar, processed and packaged. Many schoolchildren do not eat breakfast and eat snacks in the evening, resulting in low levels of regularly ingested vitamins and minerals essential for healthy tissue growth and repair. Those eating excessive amounts of these high-calorie/low-nutrient diets can become obese, with subsequent long-term development of muscular, skeletal and cardiovascular pathologies. Those pre-pubescent children eating small amounts of low-calorie foods, often with few nutrients, in order to stay slim, or who come from families on low income where food choice is limited, may also find that emotional and intellectual development deteriorates (Brown and Pollitt 1996).

Adolescence is a time of rapid development. To sustain this rate of growth the metabolism speeds up, ensuring that nutrients are processed quickly and energy released. As a result appetite increases, especially for foods with a high sugar content. It is not unusual for this age group (boys in particular) to feel the need for snacks, even before and after their main meals. 'Grazing' food can be a physiologically healthy behaviour; the stomach is given small amounts to digest at any one time in response to a desire to eat. Intake responds to a reduced blood sugar that stimulates the 'hunger centre' in the brain. McGrath and Gibney (1994) found grazing to have a favourable effect on total blood cholesterol, with a rise in high-density/low-density lipoprotein ratio occurring. However, poor management of mealtimes may result in the grazing of snacks such as chocolate, which are then favoured as a substitute for more nutritious foods.

The need for temperature control

Humans are homeothermic. They regulate their body temperature, created by their metabolic rate, in relation to their external environment. This regulation is by peripheral thermo-receptors in the skin and central thermo-receptors in the anterior hypothalamus, which monitor the temperature of the blood. As the blood passes through the hypothalamus, information is relayed to the autonomic nervous and endocrine systems for responses that return body temperature to the 'normal set point' so that enzyme activity in all the body cells can proceed.

The 'normal set point' in childhood reflects a decreasing basic metabolic rate (BMR) as the child grows. The body temperature of the three month old child is 37.5°C, whereas at thirteen years it is 36.6°C (Wong 1999). Even as the temperature regulatory mechanisms mature through childhood, babies and small children are highly susceptible to temperature fluctuations, as they produce more heat per kilogram of body weight than older children. Changes in environmental temperature, increased activity, crying, emotional upset and infections all cause a higher and more rapid increase in the younger child. The younger the child the less able he or she is to vocalise the feeling of hot or cold or to do something about it.

Children may also become too cold. Small individuals who do not have warm clothes and warm homes will not grow if the temperature of their environment is consistently low. They will use much of the energy from their food intake to generate heat (metabolic rate) and leave no spare calories for tissue growth. The smaller the child, the larger the surface area for heat loss in relation to body mass. The head of a small child is relatively larger in proportion to the rest of the body, and covering the head in a cold environment conserves heat for growth. Schoolchildren may experience a sequence of small growth spurts and at times be relatively thin with minimal body fat. At the swimming pool, for example, where children enjoy jumping in and out of the water as they play, thin children may become cold more quickly than their fatter friends who have an insulation layer beneath their skin.

The need for activity and rest

As children grow they develop more gross motor abilities and co-ordination, which allows them to further explore their world and take part in simple physical games. Exercise is essential for muscle development and tone, refinement of balance, gaining strength and endurance, and stimulating body functions and metabolic processes (Wong 1999).

Most infants enjoy being free of their clothes and allowed to kick and wriggle on a blanket on the floor, or to splash and kick in the bath. Wilsdon (1993) describes the sequential stages of motor development where the baby moves from prone to sitting to standing positions, and the need for the child to acquire these new skills by trial and error, practice and application. Children, she suggests, should be encouraged to develop a flexibility with their bodies through having the opportunity to move freely and safely.

During the school years, children are encouraged to take part in physical exercises in order to acquire timing and concentration in the more complex physical activities. They need space to run, jump, skip and climb in safety to do this, and they need the positive reinforcement of experiencing an increasingly efficient use of their body. Fitness in children can be measured in the five components of muscle strength, endurance, flexibility, body composition and cardio-respiratory endurance (American Academy of Pediatrics 1987). Improved fitness can be attained by engaging in aerobic activities for 20–25 minutes three times per week where the heart rate is maintained at 75 per cent of maximum. Children can be encouraged to be active through physical movements they enjoy, such as football and dancing. Activities that stress the skeleton against gravity will encourage uptake of calcium from the diet and thus strengthen the weight-bearing bones. School-age children enjoy competition in sport; however, their carers must be mindful of teaching proper skills appropriately, and matching activities to their physical abilities in order that excess sporting activity does not injure developing muscles and bones.

Older children who do not engage in physical pursuits, and are praised for being quiet when they play with computers and video games for long periods of time each day, are missing a critical period in their teenage years for the establishment of healthy body systems for later adult life.

Physiology knowledge in practice

Scenario

Twin sisters aged six months present, unexpectedly, at the local health visitor's clinic. Their individual body weight is low and they appear apathetic, yet they are well dressed and clean. Their young mother is anxious about them; she says that they have not been interested in food or their surroundings for about a month. What could be the reason for the twins behaving like this?

A suggested check list could include:

- Illness, such as diarrhoea or urine infection, may be evident, or there may be a more profound problem such as mild cerebral palsy.
- Small babies can be the result of a twin pregnancy, but this would not address their lack of interest in food.
- Poor breast/bottle/weaning practice may be evident on assessment. The twins may still be breast fed and thus have run out of their stores of iron. Because of this they may now be anaemic, which would explain their lethargy and failure to gain weight. They may be bottle fed and Mum is not making the bottles correctly or giving them enough to eat. The babies would then lack energy needed for growth. They may be weaning and refusing to take solid food. This also will result in lack of calories, and the result would again be lack of energy and weight gain.

Normal weight gain usually shows in a *loss* of weight: up to 10 per cent of the birth weight during the first few days of life. However, allowance must be made for the genetically large baby who has grown in the uterus of a physically small mother. This baby would, perhaps, gain weight rapidly once freed from the constrictions of the womb. The gain, then, will be approximately 200g per week until the sixteenth week, reducing to 150g until the twenty-eighth week. The 'average' infant doubles its birth weight by the fifth month, trebles it by the first year and quadruples it by the second year (McQuaid *et al.* 1996).

- Mother may be depressed. 'Baby blues' are often overlooked if the mother appears to be coping or does not take up community support systems. Father may not be helping or mother may have no social support from her family and friends, thus no one has noticed her change of behaviour and that she is neglecting her children. The mother will not 'bond' with the babies and be responsive to their demands if she is mentally unwell, so they will stop trying.

- Safety may not be assured. The twins may be very demanding to a new mother, who may abuse them. Although they are clean, they may have physical scars or be left alone for long periods of the day.

- Although the babies are well dressed at present, they may not be appropriately clothed in their own home. If the house is cold they will not thrive, as they are using the little food they get to keep warm.

- The twins may not have enough rest and sleep. They may be looked after by others during the day and/or the night. The family may live on the twentieth floor of a block of flats and have no one to help but those who live nearby. The babies may be handled a lot and not allowed to rest. They may be anxious because they have a constant stream of carers and thus are not able to relax and sleep because they do not feel safe.

- Their immunisation status may be deficient or they may be behind in their schedule. They may not have had their injec- tions until recently, and their altered condition may relate to the vaccination.

- The twins' interaction with carers may have been different before this change was noted. It would be sensible to ask what they can do now and what they could do a month ago. If they were 'term' babies they should be able to sit by this age, if propped up, and hold 'interesting' things with both hands. They should be interacting with their carers and attending to noisy and moving toys with their eyes and ears. They may not have had stimulation in this way, so their physical development may have been behind before their mother started worrying about their weight.

📖 Extend your own knowledge

Hall (1999), in the *Daily Telegraph*, reports on the Variety Club of Great Britain's 50th anniversary report, which stated that poverty in the guise of hardship, unemployment and poor housing is putting families under stress, thereby making children more vulnerable. Suicide (in the whole population) was evident in 1995, whereas in 1949 it was not in the top ten causes of death.

Q: How are child development theories useful in the context of this report, and how does government policy have a profound effect on both the physical and mental health of children in any society?

Chapter 2

The skeletal system

- Embryology
- The changing skeleton
- Growth in height
- Genetic inheritance
- Hormones of growth
- Exercise
- Nature–nurture
- Strength
- Physical play
- Body shape changes

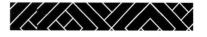

T HE DEVELOPING SKELETON changes and moulds to the forces exerted on it by the individual's muscles, other parts of the skeleton and genetic programme. This occurs not only in childhood but throughout the age span. The skeletal system is the best documented of all the systems in children; its changes and 'bone age' are recognised anatomically.

Embryology

At the end of the fourth week of foetal life, embryonic connective tissue in the region of the future skeleton shows signs of differentiation. Primitive cells become more closely packed and lay down a cartilage matrix rich in chondroitin sulphate. At six weeks of foetal life the embryonic vertebrae are forming from the mesoderm, and by the eighth week primary ossification is evident at antenatal scan. The cells round the developing cartilage form two layers: those of the outer layer change to fibroblasts, and the inner ones to cartilage and the perichondrium. Layers of cells are then added superficially as the bones grow.

Two groups of bone cells work antagonistically through life to maintain the skeleton. Osteoblasts are modified fibroblasts which have collagen fibres deposited round them. Calcium salts then accumulate here to increase bone size. Osteoclasts from the bone marrow stem cells then shape bone by removing excess material.

Ossification of many other bones also occurs in the second month of foetal life. The clavicle and bones of the skull vault ossify 'in membrane' as blood vessels penetrate the area and bring in osteoblasts and osteoclasts. Other bones ossify as the connective tissue converts to a cartilage template and then to bone. These starting points for bone ossification are called primary centres, and appear in different bones at different times.

Figure 2.1 shows the primary and secondary ossification centres.

The changing skeleton

Skeletal age is best measured at the left wrist and hand. An individual is compared to standard radiography (TW2 method). This is a score of the stage of development of the twenty bones of the wrist

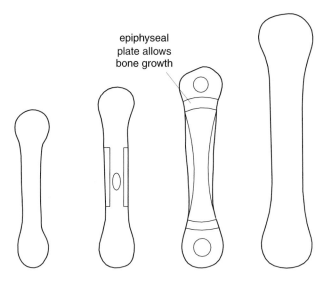

epiphyseal
plate allows
bone growth

FIGURE 2.1   Primary and secondary ossification centres

and hand. The score is relatively subjective and depends on the presence of bones and epiphyses, and the relationship of their size, shape and markings. Females are two years ahead of boys, but carpal bones are not visible under two years for either sex. The vertebral spine has two primary curves present at birth, but normally by adolescence four vertebral curves are evident: the cervical (lordotic), the thoracic (primary curve), the lumbar (lordotic) and the sacral (primary curve) (see Figure 2.2.)

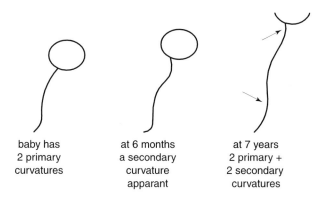

baby has
2 primary
curvatures

at 6 months
a secondary
curvature
apparant

at 7 years
2 primary +
2 secondary
curvatures

FIGURE 2.2   Development of the four vertebral curves

The baby's head shows the skull bones to be thin and the facial bones small. The jaw is small at birth with usually no teeth, but grows until puberty when adult proportions are apparent (Figure 2.3). Resuscitation in children under seven years of age demands a different technique to that of adults, as the head and neck anatomy results in relatively high positions of larynx and trachea. Small children have small facial sinuses which do not reach adult size until the age of ten/twelve years. Listen to a group at play in your local infant school and you will not be able to distinguish the individual voices of these small people who uniformly have high-pitched voices that only their mothers recognise. It will only be when they finish their growth at puberty that the genetics of their family will have been expressed. By then their faces will have developed the full number of sinuses and likeness of their parents, and their voices will show individual traits. As the sinuses increase in size, so infections are less able to become lodged in small crevices. Together with the developed ability to coordinate in order to blow one's nose, constant runny noses should become a thing of the past.

Growth in height

Growth is influenced by normal inheritance, physiological age, normal variation in nutritional status, health, hormonal status and

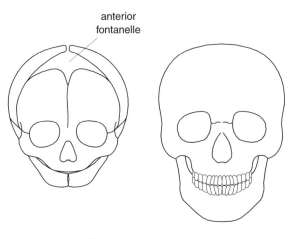

anterior
fontanelle

Skeletal system

FIGURE 2.3 Bone structure in the infant and adolescent skull

antenatal history. Voss *et al.* (1998), in the Wessex Growth Study, found that although birth weight and parental height were the major biological predictors of growth at school entry, social and environmental factors have a powerful effect. They found psychological deprivation, large families and a father who was unemployed to be the most frequent variables. Predicted height can be approximately calculated in children after the age of two years. The Child Growth Foundation charts for children from birth to eighteen (Child Growth Foundation 1994) have calculations on each chart for identifying the adult height potential. Until this time there is some readjusting of size to genetically determined growth rates. Some large babies will adjust down and some small babies will adjust up.

Genetic inheritance

The sequencing and timing of growth is influenced by the genes, and these affect different groups differently. At birth, the reason for the advanced skeletal development in females is the retarding action of the genes on the Y chromosome of the male. For example, Afro-Caribbean children grow faster in the first two years of life and their bone density is higher at all ages; males and females show different tissue growth at puberty.

Growth shows individual variation. It is distinctive of primates, and males and females show different patterns, where different parts of the body have different growth curves; for example, lymph tissue is the fastest and reproductive system the slowest in childhood (Tanner 1989). Growth shows a series of changes – specialisation of various parts of the body and alteration of body form. It includes the incidental destruction and death of cells and tissues; substitution, e.g. bone for cartilage; and modification, e.g. sexual change in the shape of the skeleton. Growth rate is different for the various body tissues, and one part may be controlled by the other, e.g. growth hormone secretion and bone length. Growth continues, e.g. the building and destruction in the moulding process of the skeleton throughout life.

Body proportions change, and there is an increase in the relative length of the legs in relation to height. There is a decreasing ratio of sitting height to stature. The body mass reduces to surface area 50 per cent from aged five years to maturity, and this is reflected in the overall reducing basic metabolic rate (BMR) in childhood. However, parents will report periods of rapid growth and periods of little growth in height – the 'Christmas tree pattern'. Peak height velocity, the maximum growth rate, is seen in the adolescent spurt.

Growth factors are usually proteins and may be produced locally – pancrine factors – or far away – endocrine factors or hormones. These growth factors act on specific protein receptors in the lipid layers of the plasma membranes of the cells to stimulate a chemical signal to the nucleus – the autocrine effect. When the cell is stimulated, amino acids are taken up into the cytoplasm to form protein, and thus growth occurs.

In childhood, growth hormone (GH) rises eight to nine times in twenty-four hours for ten to twenty minutes. Usually the bursts are at night, but there is often a short burst after entry into deep-phase sleep. GH is increased in adolescence, stimulated by the sex hormone rise. GH needs an intermediate chemical in order for it to be activated. Somatomedian is secreted by the proliferative cells in the growth plate (Figure 2.4) as well as the liver, which is the main source of this hormone.

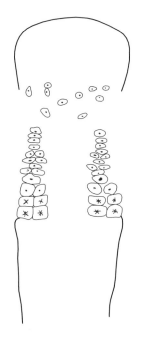

Skeletal system

FIGURE 2.4 The growth plate

Hormones of growth

Many hormones are involved in growth, some of them more involved in the developing foetus, such as prolactin, chorion gonadotrophic hormone and placenta lactogen. The hypothalamus is thought to keep the growth curve to the genetically determined pathway, and it is interesting that that a child who suffers periods of poor feeding will usually 'catch up'. The hypothalamus interacts with the pituitary to influence the whole endocrine system. Peripheral nerves also appear to play a part in exerting a nutritive or 'trophic' effect by secreting some chemical to the tissue they supply. If a hand nerve is cut, the nail does not grow well until the nerve regenerates: sensory nerves appear to effect this phenomenon more than motor nerves. Local control by chalones, chemicals which balance the cell division and differentiation phases in tissue growth, are formed by the actively dividing cells. They are also secreted by adjacent cells in the cell membranes themselves to control cell spacing. Age of tissue and its mitotic ability influence chalone secretion, thus the growing child heals quickly after injury.

Growth hormone, somatotropin, is a protein which causes most body cells to increase in size and divide. Its level in the blood is the same throughout the life span. Its major targets are the bones, cartilage, skeletal muscles and epiphyseal plates; it does not affect the brain, adrenals and gonads. The changes of adolescence rely on increased sex hormone secretion. It is an anabolic hormone which promotes protein synthesis and the use of fats for cellular fuel in order to conserve glucose. It competes for the same cell membrane receptors as insulin and is opposed by cortisol. It is stimulated to be secreted by lowering blood sugar levels, food intake, exercise and injury (especially burns). It is also affected directly by a second messenger system, the somatomedians, which are insulin-like growth factors, produced by the liver, kidneys and muscles.

GH stimulates:

- cellular uptake of amino acids from the blood and their incorporation into proteins
- uptake of sulphur needed for the synthesis of **chondroitin sulphate** into the cartilage matrix
- mobilisation of fats from adipose tissue for transport to cells, thus increasing the blood levels of fatty acids

- decreases the rate of glucose uptake and metabolism to maintain homeostatic blood glucose

It is regulated by two hypothalamic hormones with antagonistic effects. GHRH (growth hormone-releasing hormone) stimulates its release, activated by feedback blood levels of GH and somatomedian. GHIH (growth hormone-inhibiting hormone) is antagonistic to GHRH; it is a very powerful hormone which blocks other pituitary effects in the body as well as gastrointestinal and pancreatic function. These hormones have a diurnal cycle, with the steeper rise during evening sleep (Sinclair 1991).

The thyroid produces thyroxin, which accelerates the rate of cellular metabolism throughout the body. It is the regulator of growth and development; it stimulates skeletal growth and the maturation of the nervous system but inhibits that of the reproductive system. It does this by stimulating enzymes concerned with glucose oxidation, and increases metabolic rate and oxygen consumption thus increasing body heat. Thyroxin (T3 and T4) binds to the plasma proteins produced by the liver which transport it to target tissue receptors. Plasma enzymes convert T4 to T3, then remove all the thyroxin to the **mitochondria** and nucleus of the cell.

The thyroid also produces calcitonin, a hormone which antagonises parathyroid. It acts on the skeleton by inhibiting bone reabsorption and the release of ionic calcium from the bony matrix. It stimulates calcium uptake from the blood and its incorporation into the bone matrix by the osteoblasts. It increases the excretion of calcium and phosphate ions by the kidney. Raised blood calcium (over 20 per cent) stimulates its release.

The parathyroids are triggered by a decrease in blood calcium levels, and are inhibited by raised levels. Parathyroid increases ionic calcium levels by stimulating release from the skeleton, which results in the activation of the bone reabsorbing cells, the osteoclasts, which release the calcium and phosphates to the blood. It acts on the kidney tubules to reabsorb calcium ions and decrease the retention of phosphate. It increases absorption of calcium by intestinal mucosa cells. This action is enhanced by the parathyroid effect on vitamin D activation to its active form (1,25-dihydroxycholecalciferol) in the kidney.

The adrenals, activated by the hypothalamus cortisol activating hormone, stimulate the pituitary to secrete ACTH (adrenocorti-cotropic hormone), which produces three hormones from its cortex:

- *Glucocorticoids* – cortisol – influence metabolism of most body cells. Bursts occur in a pattern over the day, peaking in the morning and at its lowest level in the evening, and it is regulated by eating and physical activity. This hormone is also affected by stress, as the sympathetic nervous system overrides the inhibitory action of an elevated cortisol level on CRH release, thus ACTH continues to be released and further raises the cortisol levels. Stressed children do not grow, as they have a chronic raised metabolic rate. Cortisol also converts non-carbohydrates, i.e. fats and proteins, to glucose for energy, thus reducing the availability of these nutrients for tissue development. These high levels of glucocorticoids depress cartilage and bone formation and reduce muscle mass. Chronically stressed children will use all their nutrients for energy rather than for tissue building.
- *Mineralcorticoids* are responsible for the electrolyte composition of body fluids.
- *Androgens* stimulate metabolic processes, especially those concerned with protein synthesis and muscle growth.

The pancreas produces insulin, which facilitates glucose transfer into most cells of the body. The cells then make ATP (adenosine triphosphate, an energy source) which they use to pull amino acids from the blood to build proteins and thus support growth. Any stimulus that raises blood sugar will have this effect, such as the ingestion of food, production of adrenaline, growth hormone, thyroxin and cortisols. The production of insulin is halted by somatostatin, which is secreted by both the hypothalamus, the pancreas D cells and throughout the gastrointestinal tract. Its major affect is to inhibit insulin and glucagon local to the pancreas, where most of it is secreted. Its action is to inhibit digestive function by reducing gut motility, gastric secretion and pancreatic endocrine function and absorption at the gut mucosa. It thus paces foodstuff conversion.

Testosterone levels rise at puberty in males. This hormone effect leads to the increase in bone growth and density. The skeletal muscles also increase in size and mass. Testosterone boosts the basic metabolic rate. Energy needs are enormous at this age – ask any mother who has to feed a family of teenage boys.

Oestrogen also has an anabolic effect, particularly on the female reproductive system. The breasts grow, subcutaneous fat increases, the pelvis widens and calcium is facilitated into the skeleton. It also supports her growth spurt until levels reach high enough levels to close the epiphyseal plates and stop bone growth in length. Low oestrogen levels have been found to have a powerful effect in offsetting the positive bone mass accumulation promoted by calcium in the diet and by weight bearing exercise.

Diet calcium for bone growth

The recommended calcium intake over childhood rises with age. Infants from birth to six months require 400mg; six to twelve months, 400–700mg; one to ten years, 800–1390mg; and eleven to twenty-four years 1200–1500mg (Gallo 1996).

Exercise

Genetic factors account for 60 per cent of performance, but physical activity that stresses bones, nutritional sufficiency especially of calcium and vitamin D, hormone effect and drug use may all have a bearing on the achievement of peak bone mass. All these factors interrelate: for example, maximum physical activity with absence of normal oestrogen levels in adolescent females results in a weakened skeleton, although mechanical loading remains the pre-eminent factor for skeletal integrity (Bailey and Martin 1994). The establishment of a maximum bone density in the years of growth is vital to long-term skeletal health; 90 per cent of bone mass has been laid down by the end of puberty. This peak bone mass is difficult to determine, however, because different bones achieve their peak bone density at different times.

Nature–nurture

Genetic correlation has been found in bone mineral content, grip, strength, activity, height and triceps skin-fold thickness in three generations (Kahn *et al.* 1994). However, more recently there appears to be considerable evidence to support physical activity as the important non-inherited factor.

Changes in bone due to exercise

The key variable between skeletal loading and bone mass is the mechanical strain placed on the bone. Changes in the internal bone strain appear to activate osteoblasts, which will change the dynamic balance from bone loss to bone formation. In regular strain – repeated vigorous physical activity – there is a gain in bone formation. This increase in bone mass then reduces the load over the larger bone, and eventually balance is regained between bone loss and bone gain at the higher bone mass. However, not all activity will promote bone growth; the activity needs to be weight bearing, thus football produces good bone growth in many skeletal bones, whereas swimming and horse riding do not.

Early skeletal maturation can show an observable advantage in children being stronger and faster and with higher oxygen uptake than their 'younger' peers. Many of these children are also advanced in sexual development, as the hormones that stimulate growth in bone muscle also affect the sexual organs. This effect is most pronounced during puberty rather than before. Before puberty GH is responsible for bone and somatic growth, whereas during puberty the sex hormone effect becomes superimposed on it.

Strength

The amount of habitual physical activity effect on height is nil. Exercise has most effect on body weight where there is a decrease in body fat and increase in muscle mass and bone mineralisation, but not in bone maturation. Morris *et al.* (1997), in their study of nine to ten year olds, found that the children gained lean body mass and increased their shoulder, knee and grip strength, and also increased their bone mineral density after three thirty-minute strengthening sessions per week. Body composition has a significant influence on the physiological response to exercise as the muscle mass (motor) has to move the body fat (baggage). Small children spend most of their time in short bursts of activity which are largely anaerobic.

This activity ability increases with age, but changes are more than can be ascribed to growth and will be exercise related. Strength develops in direct relationship to neural influence, with males showing an advanced gender difference from the age of three years and increasing most during puberty under the influence of testosterone. As muscle size increases so does strength. The number of muscle fibres is fixed at birth, but as they hypertrophy they grow in size: males have 42 per cent muscle at five years and 53 per cent at seventeen years. Interestingly, there is no change in this same proportion of muscle in females as they move through puberty. Muscle structure is determined at birth by the genetic inheritance. As muscles mature their ability to contract is more efficient. Together with their growth in size, so strength increases. Resistance training for children is useful as it helps females to put down calcium and thus lessen the impact of osteoporosis in later life; it also reduces the possibility of physical injury and produces a healthier blood **lipoprotein** picture.

Activity stimulates the secretion of GH to mobilise fats for energy. In females who are very active, sex hormones are reduced as body fat reduces and muscle mass increases: thus puberty can be delayed.

Children produce a greater amount of heat relative to body mass, and they sweat less. They rely on a greater cutaneous blood flow to lose heat from their greater surface area, and small children have subcutaneous fat to insulate them. Also, a small child's head surface is 20 per cent of his or her total body surface, thus the young child adjusts slower to hot environments. Alternatively, children get hypo-thermic more quickly as they lose heat from their larger skin surface area.

Physical activity play

Pellegrini and Smith (1998) propose that physical play, although it is enjoyable, has an immediate development function for physical, cognitive and social skills. They suggest three distinct phases of physical activity.

The first is a stage of 'rhythmic stereotype' which peaks in infancy. Children at this stage strive to improve control of specific and gross motor movement patterns. This activity peaks at six months, and children can spend up to 40 per cent of their time, for example, in kicking their legs or smacking their play arch. The onset of this is controlled by neuromuscular maturation. This type of play modifies or eliminates irrelevant synapse formation. As the neurone pathways mature, infants begin to use pathways that they have developed in a more goal-directed way, for example, to manipulate toys or feeding bottles/cups.

The second stage, exercise play, can be seen in the preschool child. Here children develop their strength and endurance. They can now commence more intensive motor training as locomotion occurs. Gross motor development declines to the age of five years and only accounts for 20 per cent of their physical activity. Preschool children run, flee, wrestle, chase, jump, push and pull, lift and climb. Muscle strength, central nervous function and metabolic capacity improve skills ability and economy of movement. Exercise will have the effect of increasing muscle fibre differentiation and cerebellar synaptogenesis. The eventual outcome will be to demonstrate fine motor control. The more exercise is taken, the more endurance and strength are developed. Climbing frames, walking, riding bikes and kicking balls are all activities of play that will develop the neuromuscular pathway and remodel the skeleton. Children of this age need hourly bouts of activity each day. Interestingly, an improvement in thermoregulation is an incidental benefit.

The third stage, rough and tumble play, is seen most clearly in mid-childhood. This play also has a social animal dimension in the development of dominance function and fighting skills. From the age of six to ten years exercise play declines to 13 per cent of the child's activity. At nine to ten years, running, walking fast, games and sports, and cycling are enjoyed. Males indulge in wrestling, grappling, kicking and tumbling: this is aggressive but playful, although they will often get hurt. This activity can be seen in 4 per cent of four year olds, 7–8 per cent of six to ten year olds, 10 per cent of seven to eleven year olds, 4 per cent of eleven to thirteen year olds and 2 per cent of boys at fourteen. Children of this age are testing their strength against their peers and trying out social dominance by physical means.

Body shape changes

Parts of the body grow at different rates and have growth spurts at different times: thus the child changes radically from stage to stage of childhood (Figure 2.5). At birth the infant head is of the proportion 1:4; in the adult it is 1:8. The infant lower limbs are 15 per cent of the total body weight compared to 30 per cent in the adult. As growth proceeds, the centre of gravity moves down from the twelfth thoracic vertebra to the fifth lumbar by adult height. Thus the child's wide stance is responding to carrying a head that is twice the size of the adult, on legs that are half the length, and not necessarily responding to nappy padding. Black children, however, have relatively longer limbs, faster developing muscles, and may hold their head up, sit up and walk earlier than white children. The infant head circumference is the same as the chest; that of the abdomen is greater than both until the age of two years when the pelvic bones grow and allow abdominal contents to drop down into it. Also at this age, the neck becomes more obvious as the thorax and shoulder girdle also descend. Up to this time the ribs lie horizontal, making it difficult for small children to breathe thoracically: they persist with diaphragmatic movement. If these children suffer pain in the abdomen they may develop chest infections as they find their breathing movements compromised.

Changes in posture are related to development of the secondary

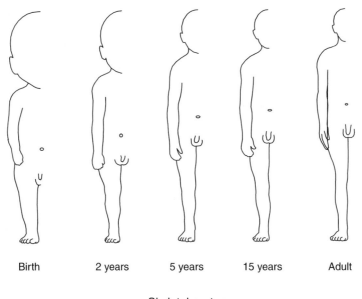

Birth　　　2 years　　　5 years　　　15 years　　　Adult

Skeletal system

FIGURE 2.5　How body proportions change with age

30

spinal curves. At four months babies pull their heads up and try to balance the head on top of the spine to fix gaze. At eight months they have the muscle strength to sit up, and the lumbar curve appears. At one year, standing against gravity needs a wide gait to balance the heavy skull, and the lumbar curve may be exaggerated, with abdomen protruding, in order to hold the upper part of the body erect until the back muscles develop the strength to maintain posture.

In the adolescent spurt the feet and hands grow first, then the calf and forearm, hips and chest, then the shoulders. Adolescent children are often accused of being clumsy; however, their bodies may have grown at such a rate that their brains have not yet reorganised spatially. The bones of the face grow, sinuses develop and the jaw drops down. Permanent teeth erupt as the 'ugly ducking' evolves. When the sex hormones take effect on the skeleton in puberty, boys' shoulders develop in response to use of their stronger pectoral muscles. Girls' pelvises becomes wider and shallower, and body fat deposits occur: the girl's shape may affect other parts of the skeleton to produce 'knock knees', flat feet and a curved thoracic spine. Towards the end of this rapid spurt the child begins to grow laterally and 'fill out'. Sheldon's three different components of physique or somatotypes – endomorph, mesomorph and ectomorph – can be recognised by the age of twenty years. These are part influenced by genetic inheritance and part by the effect of individual physical activity habit and hormone influence.

All these body changes have profound effects on each individual's psychological response throughout childhood. Toddlers who can jump in puddles will experience mastery over their world, the eight year old who can ride a bike will experience the thrill of attaining a skill, the adolescent who sees an adult body emerging will need to constantly reshape his or her identity. Physical change will also determine new social roles and expectations, and children who are too small or too big compared to their peer group will experience advantages and disadvantages in equal measure.

Physiology knowledge in practice

Scenario

Children need fresh air, sunlight, a balanced diet and exercise in order that their skeletons grow strong. Explain briefly how all these needs affect skeletal growth.

Some pointers

- Oxygen is needed by osteoblasts and osteoclasts for the release of energy to break down, remove and build bone tissue.
- Ultraviolet radiation on the skin encourages epidermal cells in the **stratum spinosum** and **stratum germinativum** to convert a steroid related to cholesterol into vitamin D. This product is absorbed, modified and released by the liver and then converted by the kidneys into calcitriol, which is needed for the absorption of calcium and phosphorus by the small intestine (Thibodeau and Patton 1999).
- Calcium gives the skeleton its strength. It is a mineral found in milk and other dairy products and bony fish. Vitamin D, not so available from sunlight in the winter months in the UK, can be found in fats such as margarine, butter and red meat.
- Exercise that is weight bearing puts stress on to the long bones, which encourages osteoclasts to lay down mineral in the bone cartilage matrix. Children should be encouraged to take part in a range of activities that includes team games, skipping, running and jumping to develop this part of their bodies, and perhaps be encouraged to walk to school each day.

📖 *Extend your own knowledge*

Mathew *et al.* (1998) described their research into the importance of bruising associated with paediatric fractures in eighty-eight healthy children from twelve to fourteen years. They found that in 91 per cent of the sample no bruising was seen, thus the pressure to break the bone must have been minimal and the bone weak, perhaps due to a temporary copper deficiency.

Q: What has copper to do with bone strength, and how might these individuals' lifestyle and physical development stages differ?

Chapter 3

The nervous system

- Brain growth embryology
- Nerve growth
- The eye and ear
- Brain growth after birth
- Fontanelles
- Nerve function
- Primitive reflexes
- Psychological maturation
- Neuromuscular control
- Sleep
- Temperature control and measurement

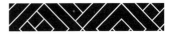

B RAIN DEVELOPMENT occurs at several stages during childhood. The critical period for brain growth appears to be during the first sixteen weeks of life. At birth, the baby's brain weighs approximately 25 per cent of its future adult weight. By the time the child is two years old the brain has increased to 75 per cent, and by six years 90 per cent of its eventual weight. This, then, indicates phenomenal growth of the central nervous system during the early years. Peripheral nerves continue to become myelinated (see **myelination**) and fine physical control appears as the child moves towards adult status. With the unique environment impinging on every waking and sleeping hour, this plastic nervous system constantly matures and changes as demands are put upon it. The nervous system coordinates and controls all body systems to a greater or lesser degree and, together with the hormones of the endocrine system, fine-tunes a delicate home-ostasis. Genetic inheritance is possibly the only restriction placed on any individual child to use their body for whatever they wish.

Brain growth embryology

The first indication of the nervous system is the neural plate, a thick-ened area of the ectoderm. It is induced to form early in the third week, and by the end of this week the neural folds have begun to fuse to the median plane to form the neural tube. This neural tube is the begin-ning of the brain and spinal cord. As the neural tube separates from the surface ectoderm cells, the neural folds form the neural crest. Ganglia of the spine, cranial and autonomic nervous system develop from the neural crest. The embryo at twenty-three days shows the hindbrain and midbrain to be formed, and the neural tube closes. In the fourth week the head folds begin to develop as the forebrain grows rapidly. In the fifth week the eye starts to grow, and cerebral hemispheres also develop from this area. The nerves of the branchial arches become the cranial nerves. Peak head breadth growth velocity occurs at thirteen post-menstrual weeks, although a relatively high velocity continues to about thirty weeks. Peak head circumference velocity occurs two to three weeks later, because the cerebellum situated at the back of the skull grows later than the cerebrum. Head volume, representing brain size, has its peak velocity at thirty weeks and growth rapidly slows after this. Different parts of the brain grow at different rates, but the hind-brain and midbrain remain the most advanced.

Figure 3.1 shows three stages of brain growth from thirty to a hundred days.

Nerve growth

The principal cells of the brain are neurones. They have long processes of two types: the single axon and one or more shorter dendrites. These neurones are the cells that carry messages throughout the body, and they occupy half of the brain volume. The neurones are supported by a group of cells called neuroglia, which provide nutrition, defence and repair of the neurons.

- *Oligodendrocytes* are responsible for myelination of axons in the central nervous system. They can myelinate several processes at any one time (see Figure 3.2).
- *Schwann cells* ensheath the axons of peripheral nerve axons. Their myeline sheath of 80 per cent lipids and 20 per cent protein insulates the nerve axon and allows rapid transmission of nerve impulse. Myelination of the nerve axons is a process that continues after birth. The nodes of Ranvier, spaces between the Schwann cells, appear constant as the nerve axon grows. As the internodal spaces elongate, the speed of transmission of the impulse increases. In general, the thicker the nerve the thicker the myeline sheath that wraps around it.
- *Satellite cells* encapsulate dorsal root and cranial nerve ganglion cells and regulate their micro-environment.

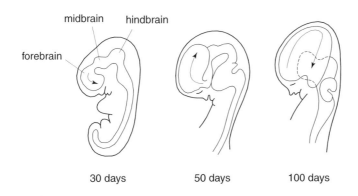

FIGURE 3.1   Brain growth, 30–100 days

- *Astrocytes* occupy interneurone spaces and connect to small blood vessels, thus allowing neurone nutrition. Their processes surround groups of synaptic endings in the central nervous system and isolate them from adjacent synapses. Their foot processes connect the blood vessels with the connective tissue at the surface of the central nervous system, which may help limit the free diffusion of substances into the central nervous system itself.
- *Microglia* transform to **phagocytes** when cells in the nervous system are damaged, and are probably derived from the circulation.
- *Ependymal cells* line the ventricles of the brain and separate the chambers for the central nervous system tissue. Many substances diffuse easily across them between the extracellular space of the brain and the cerebral spinal fluid.

The *blood/brain barrier* is an anatomical/physiological feature of the brain that separates brain parenchyma from blood. It is formed chiefly by tight junctions between capillary endothelial cells of the blood vessels. These cerebral capillaries have no fenestrations or pores, and are thought to be responsible for the selective nature of the blood/brain barrier when mature. (Berne and Levy 1996; Mera 1997). Histological evidence shows astrocyte processes, capillary endothelium and neurone membranes to be closely associated. The

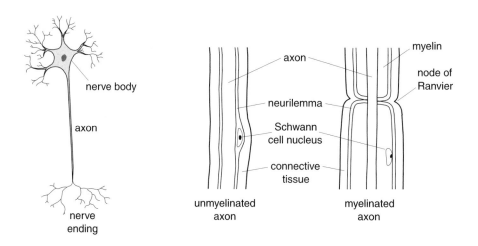

FIGURE 3.2 Axon myelination

blood/brain barrier is a term used to describe its function, based on observations that facilitated diffusion of glucose and passive diffusion of water and carbon dioxide is allowed, but it is impermeable to protein and does not permit passage of many active substances. The functional importance of this barrier is more to do with the endothelial cells stopping substances moving out of the central nervous system than stopping substances such as neurotoxins entering. However, in the foetus and newborn, it is indiscriminately permeable, allowing passage of protein and other large and small molecules to pass freely between the cerebral vessels and the brain. Harmful substances such as lead have been found to accumulate in certain individuals exposed to this metal; most ions such as sodium and potassium are regulated in order not to disrupt the transmission of nerve impulses. The blood/brain barrier functions to exclude substances that are of low solubility in lipid, such as organic acids, highly ionized polar compounds, large molecules and substances not transported by specific carrier-mediated transport systems. These include albumin and substances bound to albumin such as bilirubin, many hormones and drugs, organic and inorganic toxins. Because the young child does not have mature function, osmotic changes and free bilirubin in the blood, for example, will allow water and bilirubin to enter and damage brain tissue in abnormal circumstances (Nowak and Handford 1994). Conditions that cause cerebrovascular dilation such as hypertension, hypercapnia, hypoxia and acidosis disrupt the blood/brain barrier. Hyperosmotic fluids which cause shrinkage of vascular endothelium and thus widen the vascular junctions also interfere with normal protective function (Wong 1999).

Growth in nerve cell size occurs as the early embryonic neurones absorb nutrients and fluids from their environment. Once formed, a nerve cell can increase in mass up to 200,000 times, most of the addition being to the processes of the cells. Each of these processes may come to contain as much as a thousand times the amount of material contained in the cell body. The diameter of the myelinated nerve cells in peripheral nerve trunks increases considerably; the nerve cells contain much RNA (ribonucleic acid), which is used to form cytoplasm to be pushed into rapidly growing dendrites. By eighteen weeks' gestation, most of the neurons' nuclei are formed in the cerebrum, but neuroglial cells continue to be produced here up to two years of age. Neuroglial cells in the cerebellum, on the other hand, begin to form earlier at fifteen weeks and continue to be formed until fifteen months after birth. By six months' gestation, nerve cells are growing in size rather than dividing, and there is a huge increase in the cytoplasm that allows interconnections to be made. Ramification and myelination of their processes occurs.

In the skin there are marked changes in the neural pattern. During the third month of intra-uterine life the epidermis begins to stratify, and it is immediately invaded by branches from the cutaneous plexus of nerves. As the organised endings appear in the skin, the intra-epidermal fibres and endings withdraw, so that after birth only a few remain. In the dermis the organised sensory endings, such as the Meissner corpuscles, are closely packed together but as the skin grows they become thinned out. Thus the tiny baby has acute skin sensation, but as the child grows the skin receptors become more widely spaced, particularly over the dorsal surface of the body.

The eye

The neural parts of the eye are evident at the fourth week after conception, when optic grooves develop in the neural folds at the cranial end of the embryo. Eyelids develop from the folds of the surface ectoderm and fuse at the eighth week of foetal life. They then remain closed until about week twenty-six of gestation (Matsumura and England 1992).

The cells of the visual area of the cortex have their peak burst of development in the period between twenty-eight and thirty-two weeks' gestation. The 'visual analyser' starts to myelinate shortly before birth and completes rapidly by the tenth week after birth to cope with visual stimuli. The cornea and lens of the eye will cast an image of the environment on the photoreceptors of the retina, each of which will respond to the intensity of the light that falls on it. A mosaic pattern is formed which passes via the optic nerves, optic chiasma and thalamus to the visual cortex in the occipital lobe of the cerebrum. Several other regions of the brain, including the hypothalamus and brain stem, will also receive visual information. These other regions help regulate activity during the day/night cycle, coordinate eye and head movements, control attention to visual stimuli and regulate the size of the pupils (Carlson 1998). Some mothers report their baby to have a day/night cycle in the third trimester of pregnancy; perhaps the light-sensitive retina begins to signal a light/dark rhythm at this time.

Children need to focus light on to the central part of the retina, the fovea, for the cones to develop. There seems to be a critical time for this development, about the age of three to four years, otherwise the child will never be able to see distinctly. The eyeball is at first too short for its lens, so most infants have about 1 dioptre of long-sightedness. As it grows, the eyeball becomes longer but the converging power of the cornea and lens reduces, thus cancelling out the refractive error of the newborn. One needs to hold small babies at a distance of about twenty centimetres when talking to them, but by six months of age they can see the feeding bottle and parent from across a room. The lens then continues to grow throughout life: at fourteen years it is of adult size, but by sixty years it is one-third bigger than the young adult of twenty years.

The ear

The outer ear, the auricle, grows at the same rate as the body developing from the dorsal portion of the branchial groove. The inner ear, the middle ear cavity and the drum are of almost adult size at birth. The inner ear develops as an otic pit either side of the hindbrain early in the fourth week after conception, and is complete by the eighth week of embryonic life. The middle ear develops from the first pharyngeal pouch and soon envelopes the middle ear bones which develop from the first and second branchial arches. The fibres of the 'acoustic analyser' (Carlson 1998) begin to myelinate at the sixth month of foetal life but do not complete until the end of the fourth year, possibly in relation to the development of language. In the womb babies are sensitive to sounds from their mothers' viscera. Sound waves are transmitted to the inner ear, and via the auditory nerve to the medulla. Neurones synapse here to the auditory cortex in the temporal lobe, with the stimulus mainly going to the same hemisphere as the ear receiving the sound. However, stimuli also go to the cerebellum and reticular formation. Babies can detect pitch, loudness and timbre of sound, and also location and changes in complex sounds. New babies appear well programmed to listen to their mothers' voice and be soothed by it. The other functions of the ear are to control posture, head movement and eye movement.

Information from this part of the ear is received in the medulla which relays it to the cerebellum, spinal cord, pons and temporal cortex.

Birth onwards

The new baby can cry, suck, swallow, sneeze, move her eyes, defecate and micturate, taste and smell. She can feel pain and has a powerful grasp. She faces two main challenges: to learn about her environment and to stand upright against gravity.

The brain

The two hemispheres of the human brain are not mirror images of each other; the upper surface of the temporal lobe and the whole occipital region is larger on the left side than on the right. The left area receives, processes and is concerned with producing language. The right hemisphere processes spatial information both visual and tactile. There is some debate as to whether this difference is part of the difference between the brains of males and females.

In the newborn, the brain is 10–12 per cent of body weight and doubles in the first year of life. It continues this growth spurt begun in mid-pregnancy. By two years the nerve **dendrites** will have been pruned of the redundant pathways (Bee 1992).

To accommodate this growth the sutures between the skull bones are not yet fused at birth, and there are two openings in the skull which can be easily felt. The anterior fontanelle, which can be felt in the midline of the skull above the brow, closes gradually in the first eighteen months of life, while the smaller posterior fontanelle, again in the midline but towards the back of the baby's head, is normally closed by the age of six weeks. The normal fontanelle is flat but may pulsate with the heartbeat or bulge when the baby coughs or strains. It may feel soft or slightly springy from the support of the layer of the cerebral spinal fluid, which circulates under the arachnoid membrane to cushion and protect the delicate brain. If the fontenelle appears depressed the child may be dehydrated. If the fontanelle bulges it may indicate that the flow of cerebral spinal fluid is impeded, such as in the child with hydrocephalus or meningitis.

The brain volume is reflected in head circumference measured at the greatest circumference from the top of the eyebrows and pinna of the ears to the occipital prominence of the skull. At birth the head circumference exceeds the chest circumference by 2–3cm, at one to two years it equals the chest circumference, but during childhood the chest circumference eventually exceeds the head circumference by 5–7cm (Wong 1996).

The most active parts of the brain at birth (see Figure 3.3) are the sensori-motor cortex, the thalamus, the brain stem and the cerebellum. All the major surface features of the cerebral hemispheres are present at birth, but the cerebral cortex is only half its adult thickness. The spinal cord is about 15–18cm long, with its lower end opposite either the second or third lumbar vertebra. The spinal cord does not grow as much as the vertebral canal and therefore appears to rise up as the child grows in length. All the major sensory tracts are fairly well myelinated, but the motor tracts less so. However, the local reflexes related to swallowing and sucking appear before birth and have their nerve pathways well myelinated.

The nerves

At birth much of the nerve tissue still has little myeline insulation;

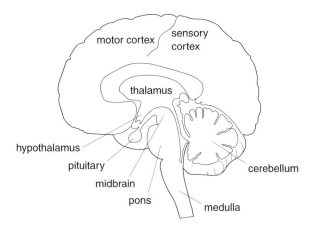

FIGURE 3.3   The most active parts of the brain at birth

thus the rate of nerve transmission is slower than the adult and the movement is less efficient. This control of movement improves as the myeline increases and the child interacts with the environment. Although there is a wide range of normal movements, the sequence of development shows the same steps. First is the cephalocaudal, or head-to-toe development as the child shows the ability to control the head and face before the lower limbs. Development is also prox-imodistal where the development of the midline occurs before that of the extremities: the baby controls the arm before the fingers. The child controls the general before the specific: the arm-waving motion is gained before the finer control of manipulating a toy. At all ages balance and the ability to control the head, trunk and limbs is important; later the gait and the ability to control the body in space is a necessary milestone. Babies' levels of consciousness can be assessed by their level of activity and interest in the environment and their interaction with people.

Motor development in the baby reflects the neuromuscular matu-ration and is related to the rapid growth of the brain at this time. The association, noticeable in the infant stage, may be related to the unique growth spurt of the cerebellum. This controls the develop-ment and maintenance of neuromuscular coordination, balance and muscle tone. Whereas in the rest of the brain there is a spurt in the number of neuroglial cells, the cerebellum starts its spurt later than the cerebrum and brain stem but completes it earlier. The cerebrum and brain stem begin their growth spurt at about mid-pregnancy, whereas the cerebellum starts a month or two before term. By eighteen months of age the estimated cell count of the cerebellum has reached adult levels, whereas the cerebrum and brain stem have achieved only 60 per cent. It is during this time that the infant develops the postural control and balance needed for walking.

Reflexes

Young babies at birth are equipped with a number of primitive instinctive movements which assist them to survive. These motor responses are extensions of those established during foetal life. These patterns take the form of reflexes that are either present at birth or appear in infancy. Some of the reflexes are simple and are mediated at the spinal cord level; others are more complex and require the integration of brain centres, the labyrinths and other developing nervous centres.

- Primitive reflexes associated with feeding such as the rooting, sucking and tongue retrusion reflex are well developed at birth. One can elicit this response by stroking the baby's cheek so he or she turns the head towards this stimulus.
- The corneal and blinking reflexes are strong and can be seen when the baby is carried in a wind or faced towards the sun.
- The palmar grasp is a flexor response and is characterised by a relatively strong flexion of the palm and fingers without thumb opposition.
- The planter reflex also shows the same strong response as the palmar grasp on the inferior aspect of the foot.
- The Moro reflex, where the startled child will fling his or her arms symmetrically apart and then bring them together again, is the most consistent primitive developmental milestone between birth and three months. The extensor response can be demonstrated by any sudden movement of the neck region. The infant reacts with extension and abduction of the extremities and a noticeable tremor of the hands and feet.
- The startle reflex, which is similar to the Moro, is stimulated by a loud unexpected noise, and the baby responds as to the Moro response but with flexion rather than abduction of the extremities.

A second set of reflexes, the locomotor reflexes, resemble later voluntary movements that will allow the child to move through space. These include creeping, standing, stepping and swimming. These movements do not involve voluntary control at first, and indicate a lack of inhibition of the segmental apparatus of the nervous system. As this matures in infancy and childhood, the inhibitory functions of the cerebral cortex begin to operate, and these reflex movements gradually diminish and are integrated into voluntary patterns. There is much variation in these reflex responses in children as well as within the same child – they may change with behavioural states. However, their presence or absence is indicative of normal nervous system development and vital to later ability to walk, run and jump.

The third group of reflexes in the newborn are the postural reflexes. One of these is the tonic neck reflex. This develops in the first few months of life. When the baby's head is turned to one side he or she responds with an increased muscle tone and extension of both the arm and the leg of the side to which the face is turned, and by the flexion of the arm and leg of the opposite side. Another postural reflex, the righting reflex, facilitates maintenance of the relationship between the head and other body parts. The third postural reflex, the labyrinthine reflex, orientates the body relative to the force of gravity. These postural reflexes begin to emerge at about three months and increase in intensity throughout infancy. Their function is to help the baby maintain or regain its balance against gravity when disturbed (Malina and Bouchard 1991).

It appears that the primitive reflexes disappear as functional abilities such as turning towards sound, gazing at moving objects, reaching under conscious control for attractive objects, increased manipulative control and weight bearing through legs allow mobility to develop (McQuaid *et al.* 1996)

Psychological maturation

Maturation of psychological awareness develops from a self-centred absorption to the recognition of parent and then peers. Mental age may be measured by performance tests such as the Stanford Binet Test and the Wechsler scale, which take cognisance of maths, verbal and logic ability as well as other capacities. An Intelligence Quotient (IQ) can be devised by scoring children's mental age as a percentage of their chronological age; thus a child of mental age twelve who is ten years old would have an IQ of 120. In the UK those with an IQ of 120 are considered capable of a university education and those who score 60 or below are offered 'special' schooling. Personality and other psychological developments change as the nervous system interacts with a unique environment for every child. Mind and physical brain are both separate and linked, but mind, for now, is outside the remit of this book.

Neuromuscular control

Two clear gradients occur in the cerebral cortex during the first two years after birth, the first to do with general functional areas (see Figure 3.4) and the second to do with body location.

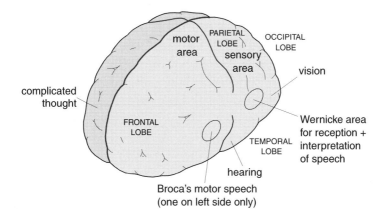

FIGURE 3.4   General functional areas in the cerebral cortex

General functional areas

- The most advanced part of the cortex is the primary motor area located in the pre-central gyrus, the cells which initiate movement.
- The second area to develop is the primary sensory area in the post-central gyrus where nerve fibres mediate the sense of touch.
- The third area to develop is the primary visual area in the occipital lobe where nerve paths from the retina end.
- The fourth area to develop is the primary auditory area in the temporal lobe.

All the association areas lag behind the primary areas, but gradually a wave of maturation moves out from the primary centres:

- In the motor area control of arm and upper trunk, which develops ahead of those controlling the leg.
- In the leg movement, which can take at least two years to develop fully. A number of tracts will not have completed their myelination even after four years of life.
- In the reticular formation, concerned with the maintenance of

47

attention and consciousness, which continues to be myelinated until puberty.

- In the cerebrum near the midline, which is suggested to be related to the development of hormonal and metabolic activity related to reproductive behaviour (Yakovlev 1967, cited in Tanner 1989).

Body location

During the first two years of life the child gradually attains postural, locomotor and prehensile control. Motor development is viewed as representing neuromuscular maturation. However, motor development is a plastic process, and variation in the sequence, timing and rate of development is most likely to relate to a variety of biological (genetic, body size and composition) and environmental (rearing atmosphere, play opportunities and objects) factors.

Walking is a major task for the two year old. There has to be prior control of the head, upper trunk and upper limbs, then the control of the entire trunk, in the development of sitting unaided. Creeping and crawling is then followed by standing with and without support. This advanced ability is usually achieved by fifteen months. A mature walking pattern is usually achieved by four years of age, and the acquisition of fundamental motor skills progresses rapidly, these being normally attained by 60 per cent of six to seven year olds.

Boys tend to attain the skill of throwing and kicking earlier than girls, but girls tend to hop and skip earlier than boys. Fundamental motor skills are defined by Malina and Bouchard (1991) as climbing, jumping, hopping, skipping, galloping, throwing and catching. It is interesting that children may achieve a mature skill, only to regress while another motor skill is learnt, and then to regain that particular mature skill later.

Sleep

Sleep is a protective behaviour in all organisms. Some authors say that it allows for repair and recovery of tissues following activity; others say that it has evolved from a time when humans needed to keep relatively motionless at times when moving around would be dangerous or simply wasteful of energy (Goodale 1994). Asleep, children show two very different cyclical phases, and even in the waking state they show these cyclical patterns in high- and low-activity levels.

Figure 3.5 shows the 'sleep centres' in the brain.

Sleep is induced by complex neuro-chemical reactions arising in the tissues of the brain stem known as the reticular formation and mediated by neurotransmitters such as serotonin and noradrenaline. Superimposed on this mechanism are circadian rhythms, which are thought to be controlled by the pineal gland, and external clues such as light and dark (Hodgson 1991).

Slow wave sleep (non-REM) is promoted by the Raphé system, and REM (Rapid Eye Movement) sleep is promoted as the activity of neurones in the locus coeruleus increase. The former state is characterised by slow brain waves and movement of body position. Some children are very 'restless' at night in this type of sleep and throw off their covers or fall out of bed. The latter state is quite complex, a paradox in fact, because the brain appears to be active and the eyes move under their lids while the body lies very still. Goodale (1994) suggests that this REM sleep is increased in infants

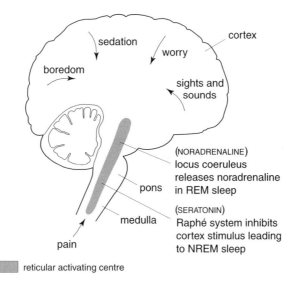

FIGURE 3.5 The 'sleep centres' in the brain

and young children as they are learning a lot about their world at a rapid rate, thus they must organise and integrate this with existing memories. He also suggests that children who are intellectually gifted seem to spend more time in this type of sleep than other children, and that retarded children engage in it less. However, those who are deprived of sleep appear to be able to survive adequately, but lack of sleep may have more subtle effects on the child's development, especially if it interferes with schooling.

As children mature, the quantity and quality of sleep changes. Family influences, social expectations and cultural variations affect the amount of sleep a child experiences. The length of time a child sleeps decreases throughout childhood. Newborn babies sleep for much of the time not occupied with feeding; interestingly, the time intervals are longer the larger the baby is, as the stomach holds more feed. During the latter part of the first year the baby may sleep all night and also have naps during the day. By the age of two years many children will only have a short daytime nap and, by the age of three years, most children will not sleep during the day except in cultures where a siesta is customary. From four to ten years the period of night-time sleep shortens slightly but increases again during puberty (Campbell and Glasper 1995).

Sleep can be disrupted by many changes in routine, such as sleeping in another bed or being put to bed by another carer. Many researchers have documented these problems and suggested ways to overcome resistance at bedtime. Kerr *et al.* (1996) suggested that sleep problems are common in preschool children, and that 22 per cent of nine month olds have difficulty settling, with 42 per cent waking at night. The authors developed an intervention programme from their study that showed settling difficulties and night waking could be helped by supporting the parent. They were, however, clear that sleep problems are multifactoral and may include the environmental effects of overcrowding, poverty and maternal mental health. Atkinson *et al.* (1995) would suggest also that aspects of the child's individual temperament should be considered when assessing this complex problem of a child who will not go to sleep. Mindell *et al.* (1994) support Kerr *et al.*'s view that sleep behaviour is a common problem: they found that 25 per cent of all children under sixteen years experience some kind of sleep disturbance. Sleep talking, nightmares, waking at night, trouble with falling asleep, enuresis, bruxism, sleep rocking and night terrors were all reported.

Yarcheski and Mahon (1994) found that middle adolescents experienced the highest level of sleep disturbance, such as sleep latency, mid-sleep waking and movement during sleep, and suggested that this reflected the intense emotional period of such children's lives as they struggle for independence. They suggested that reports from girls that they benefited less from their sleep were perhaps due to their hormonal changes and their intuitive reporting of moodiness and level of fatigue. All adolescents showed a higher level of sleep supplementation in the mornings or early evenings; however, the total time in twenty-four hours for all teenagers was consistently in the range 8.0–7.8 hours. The reasons they found for these changes in sleep patterns were expanding social opportunities, academic demands, involvement in part-time jobs and an increased access to alcohol and drugs. Perhaps an investigation into the sleep patterns of the adolescent would improve the professional's understanding of some of this age group's special problems and health needs.

Temperature control

The maintenance of body temperature is mainly coordinated by the hypothalamus, which contains large numbers of heat-sensitive neurones. It is an important homeostatic mechanism which allows the body enzymes to work efficiently. In response to a change in temperature, the peripheral thermoreceptors transmit signals to the hypothalamus, where they are integrated with the receptor signals from the preoptic area of the brain.

Heat is created by:

- Metabolism in the liver, skeletal muscles and other chemical actions. Metabolism releases chemical energy from the covalent bonds of hydrogen compounds, fat and carbohydrates, and the energy that is not used for cell activity is lost as heat.
- Shivering, which is involuntary and spasmotic contraction and relaxation of skeletal muscles. This occurs when the environmental or core temperatures drop.
- The pilomotor reflex, which makes hair on the skin stand up due to contraction of the pilomotor muscles in the hair follicles (R. Watson 1998).

When infants are placed in a cool environment, metabolic activities occur that can result in hypoglycaemia, elevated serum bilirubin, metabolic acidosis and increased metabolic rate. When heat loss begins, non-shivering thermogenesis (NST) is triggered by thermoreceptors in the subcutaneous tissue, hypothalamus and spinal cord. This may begin within the first four hours after birth from the 'cold stress' of delivery. Noradrenaline binds to brown adipocyte beta-1-adrenoreceptors and triggers cellular respiration through the increase of cyclic adenosine monophosphate (cAMP). Brown fat accounts for 4 per cent of the new baby's fat mass and is found around the kidney and adrenal, muscles and blood vessels of the neck, in the mediastinum and the scapular and axillae. It is deposited between weeks twenty-six to thirty of gestation but is insufficient in quantity to be useful until week thirty-six. Brown fat metabolism triggers lipolysis and heat production. Vasodilation from heat production then results in 25 per cent of the cardiac output flowing through these dilated vessels and thus maintains core temperature. During this process oxygen is used by brown fat at three times the rate of other body tissues, and the increased breakdown of triglycerides to non-esterified free fatty acids results in a metabolic acidosis. These fat metabolites compete with the bilirubin for albumin sites, and thus the bilirubin levels will rise. If available glucose is used at this higher rate and replacement of energy from food not addressed, the infant will eventually become hypo-glycaemic and convulse as the brain is deprived of sugar. In measuring temperature by axilla in the term baby, one may assume the baby is warm whereas the infant is perhaps too cold. It is recommended to take both tympanic (core) and axilla (shell) temperature in the infant if the professional is in doubt (Bliss-Holtz 1993).

Heat is lost

- through contact with a cooler environment
- by vasodilation, where the peripheral blood vessels dilate due to inhibition of the sympathetic centres in the posterior hypothalamus
- by sweating, where the preoptic area in the anterior hypothalamus is stimulated causing secretion of water to the skin surface for evaporation
- by a decrease in heat-producing activity (Edwards 1998)

Thus temperature measurement in children is important to clarify the observed characteristics of changes from normal. The immature brain has a more labile homeostatic control than the adult. Under five years of age, children's brains become irritated by overheating. Parents and carers may observe changes in skin colour, posture, fluid intake and output, and level of activity and behaviour. However, as temperature has a circadian rhythm, a reading of 37.5°C at 14.00 hours will not necessarily indicate a fever, but taken at 02.00 hours it may (Harrison 1998). Normal temperature of an infant at night may be 36.0°C and rise to 37.8°C if active in the day, giving a normal mean of 36.9°C.

There are many tools on the market today to measure temperature:

- The typanic membrane infra red device is favoured in hospitals as it is quick to use and reflects the blood supply servicing the hypothalamus, thus giving a core reading. However, it is expensive and the earpiece needs to be the correct size for the size of the child. It is not accurate if the eardrum is occluded by cerumen (O'Toole 1998).
- An axilla reading taken with an electronic probe is easy to access and safe, but can give a false reading if the child is sweating or has a large layer of insulating fat. A small child can squirm and dislodge this type of probe from the skin surface.
- The mercury/glass clinical thermometer used in the mouth is not considered safe for many children, as they cannot hold it correctly with the mercury reservoir under the tongue near the lingual artery.
- Disposable thermometers are popular with families as they pose no safety threat, are reasonably accurate and are easily available from the high street pharmacy.

Physiology knowledge in practice

Scenario

Children in the six to seventeen year age-band receive little touch. The younger child is being encouraged to grow up and not act like a baby, and the teenager may find it embarrassing or threatening. Also, fathers may see touching their children as a taboo in contemporary society (S. Watson 1998). How could massage be beneficial in soothing a child?

Some pointers

- There are four categories of touch, the first being instrumental, where there is deliberate physical contact. The second, expressive, is seen in the spontaneous hug that teenagers hate. The third is therapeutic touch, where there is a transfer of energy with the intention to heal. The fourth is systemic touch, which is an intentional touch aimed to enhance the receiver's well-being. It is this last type of touch that is synonymous with massage (Simms 1986, cited in S. Watson 1998).
- The benefit of massage is to promote relaxation: this relieves muscle tension.
- The cutaneous sensory information is perceived by kinesthetic receptors in the skin. These respond to constant mechanical pressure. Their axons share nervous pathways with the motor neurone fibres of muscles to the spinal ganglia.
- Impulses move, under constant mechanical pressure stimulation, to the thalamus and somatosensory cortex of the brain.
- The brain cortex responds by stimulating impulses to the amygdala and hypothalamus: enkephalins are produced which are opiate-like chemicals produced by the central nervous system.
- The medulla is then activated to stimulate the spinal dorsal horn neurones which inhibit noxious stimuli, e.g. muscle tension signals.
- Other parts of the brain are also activated, such as the hypothalamus, which controls the autonomic nervous system and endocrine system (Carlson 1998).

Extend your own knowledge

Krueger *et al.* (1998) in their article on the humoral regulation of sleep, suggest that one of the humoral mechanisms that control sleep is growth hormone-releasing hormone (GHRH). They showed that injections of this chemical increased the length of time in non-REM sleep and electroencephalogram (EEG) slow-wave activity.

Q: Why don't anxious children grow?

Chapter 4

The cardiovascular system

- Heart embryology
- Foetal heart circulation
- Heart circulation after birth
- Changes in circulation in childhood
- Exercise and the heart
- Blood pressure and exercise
- Children's blood
- Common blood tests
- Routine diet supplement

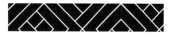

THE NORMAL RESTING metabolism needs adequate body perfusion of blood. The rising energy requirements in children as they grow must be matched by similar improvements in cardiac output. Basic metabolic rate (BMR), related to the increasing body mass and relative decrease of surface area, becomes increasingly inversely related to body size. Resting BMR must relate to cardiac output for health.

Heart embryology

In the fourth week after conception a pair of angioblastic cords develop from the mesoderm to form a pair of endocardial tubes, which then fuse to form the primitive heart tube. This starts to beat on day twenty-two, shunting blood round the embryo by day twenty-four. Between weeks five and eight this tube remodels to transform into four chambers. In the fifth week septi grow to separate the right and left atria, also the valves between the atria and septi form. The right atrial fibre tract develops to form the heart pacemaker, as up to this time the heart has 'beaten' due to myogenic stimulus as the blood flowed through tubes whose walls contain myocytes enervated by the autonomic nervous system. The ventricles are separated by the eighth week; this last intricate remoulding is vital, with most common defects at birth being found here.

Starting from day seventeen, spaces occur in the splanchnic mesoderm and blood vessels begin to arise from the yolk sac wall 'blood islands' that interconnect and develop into the endothelium of the primitive blood and lymph circulation. Valves in veins are present at six months of foetal life. Lymphatic channels arise in the fifth embryonic week (Larsen 1993). Primitive blood cells arise within the yolk sac and the extraembryonic mesoderm associated with the chorion (Marieb 1997). Blood cell production on day eighteen switches from the yolk sac to the liver, spleen, thymus and finally the bone marrow.

Foetal heart circulation

Oxygenation occurs in the placenta for the foetus which is an inefficient oxygenation system. Thus the foetus is always hypoxic with an aortic arterial oxygenation saturation of 60–70 per cent. To maintain adequate oxygen delivery, foetal cardiac output is thus higher at

44–500ml/kg/min than in the neonate, in order to maintain blood supply to the foetal brain. In the foetal circulation oxygenated blood enters the body through the left umbilical vein. It then mixes a small volume of deoxygenated blood that is returning from the portal system, legs and lower body trunk in the inferior vena cava. The flow moves up to the right atrium, where it then flows to the left atrium through the *foramen ovale* in a distinct stream alongside the deoxy-genated blood from the superior vena cava, draining blood from the head and upper trunk (Figure 4.1). Here, there is a little mixing with the small amount of blood that returns, having circulated to nourish the developing pulmonary tissue before it returns via the pulmonary veins. Pulmonary resistance is very high, as the foetal lung fields are filled with fluid so that the hypoxic alveoli stimulate pulmonary vessel vasoconstriction. Most of the returning superior vena cava blood moves into the right ventricle, which would then normally flow into the lungs. In the foetus only some of this blood then moves up the pulmonary artery towards the lungs; the rest is diverted into the *ductus arteriosus* which bypasses the lungs to the descending aorta. The still well-oxygenated blood is then propelled to the foetus' body tissues, which offer little vascular resistance, via the aorta, before returning to the placenta via the umbilical artery for oxygenation. Figure 4.2 shows the scheme of foetal circulation.

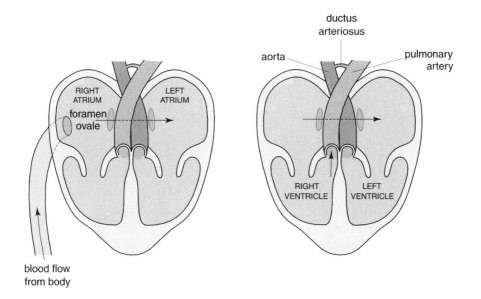

FIGURE 4.1   Foramen ovale and ductus arteriosos

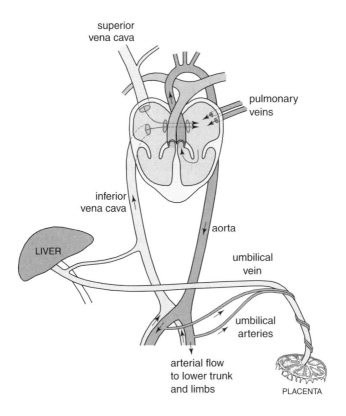

FIGURE 4.2 Foetal circulation

One of the factors that favours oxygen diffusion across the placenta to the developing foetus is that the haemoglobin, type f, produced *in utero* is not affected by the 2,3DPG which is present in the adult red cells to induce offloading to tissues. Therefore, the foetal haemoglobin oxygen curve shows slightly greater oxygen affinity than does that of the mother. Also the haemoglobin concentration in the foetal blood is high, 200g/l, so the foetus' arterial blood has nearly the same oxygen concentration as that of its mother, even though its arterial oxygen pressure is less than 40mm mercury (Staub 1996).

Circulation changes in the heart at birth

At birth the heart occupies 40 per cent of the lung fields (30 per cent in adults). Changes in the foetal circulation at birth occur as babies start to depend on their lungs for oxygen rather than the mother's placenta.

The **Apgar score** taken at one minute and five minutes after birth is scored for a pulse which is either absent (0 points), or lower than 100 (1 point) or above 100 (2 points). These scores are added to scores from other critical measurements (linked to respiratory, muscular skeletal and nervous systems) and together they predict satisfactory survival of the infant. However, the baby may look blue at the extremities for a few hours after birth (Table 4.1).

At birth when the infant takes its first breath, the alveoli in the lungs fill with air and the constricted pulmonary vessels open to allow more blood to flow to the lungs. At the same time umbilical flow is halted. The pressure changes, and reduction of prostaglandins that maintained the pregnancy causes the *ductus arteriosis* and *foramen ovale* to close. This happens over the first ten to fifteen hours of extra-uterine life in the term baby. Thus the newborn baby may exhibit a soft systolic murmur which will disappear as the cardiac circulation adapts to pressure changes in circulation. Oxygen consumption doubles from 7–8ml/kg/min to 15–18ml/kg/min. Thus a corresponding ventricular output is seen. Oxygen demand remains high, and anything that increases oxygen demand, e.g. cold or sepsis, will stress the baby's heart. At eight weeks oxygen consumption drops by 50 per cent. Hepatic flow

TABLE 4.1 Apgar score sheet

Score	0	1	2
Heart rate	Absent	<100 beats/min	>100 beats/min
Respiratory effort	Absent	Gasping/irregular	Regular/strong cry
Muscle tone	Flaccid	Some flexion of limbs	Well flexed/active
Reflex irritability	None	Grimace	Cry/cough
Colour	Pale/blue	Body pink/extremities blue	Pink

Source: Lissauer and Clayden 1997

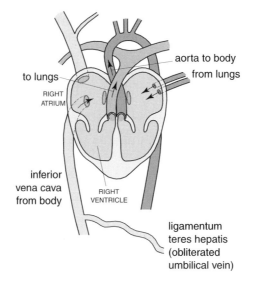

FIGURE 4.3 Circulation after birth

ensured by the umbilical vein, and also kept patent by prostaglandins in the foetus, is taken over by the portal system within a few days after birth.

Figure 4.3 illustrates circulation after birth.

Changes in the cardiovascular system in childhood

The mass of the heart as a ratio of the body mass is high in babies but reduces as childhood progresses. There is a 20 per cent decline from three to fifteen years. The left ventricle mass closely relates to body surface area. La Place's law requires that a rise in blood pressure with age is matched by a proportionately greater ratio of wall thickness to chamber dimensions to maintain constant wall stress. Over childhood cardiac muscle fibres increase seven times in size, with cardiac blood vessels increasing in number to supply them; however, small babies have greater myocardial contractility than older children. Although children's cardiac responses to exercise are poorly researched due to ethical considerations, Armstrong and Welsman (1997) consider the available results to be unequivocal. Cardiac scope rises with age, but children's and adolescents' cardiac outputs are lower than those of adults at any given level of oxygen uptake.

Cardiac output is related to heart rate and stroke volume (Table 4.2). Children's smaller hearts (stroke volume) beat faster (rate) to oxygenate their body tissues. Resting stroke volume is related to body weight, but this is influenced by body composition, for example, lean body mass. Children of different sizes have different normal ranges of cardiac output, thus the cardiac index (CI) is often used for them:

CI = CO divided by body surface in metres squared (normal is 3.5–4.5l/min/m^2 of body surface)

Any increase in normal rate, however, does not improve cardiac function. With over 200–220 beats/min in infants and 160–180 beats/min in children, one would see a ventricular diastolic filling time and coronary artery perfusion time reduced, leading to a fall in stroke volume and cardiac output. In fact, **transient bradicardia** may then occur which leads to a fall in systemic perfusion; the child becomes mottled and pale in colour; peripheral vasoconstriction occurs; peripheral extremities become cool; there is delayed capillary refill; decreased urine output is seen, and a metabolic acidosis is evident. Interestingly, arterial systolic blood pressure may remain normal as the result of arterial constriction.

Fat children's cardiac output may, therefore, be underestimated. Obesity in children cannot be well defined, due to their total body water and reduced bone density. Body fat to skin fat ratio is higher anyway in children. Heart rate falls in childhood (Table 4.3), and from nine years gender effects are also seen. (Basal rates are those

TABLE 4.2 Normal paediatric cardiac output (CO):stroke volume (SV)

Age	Pulse	CO l/min	SV
Newborn	145	0.8–1.0	5
6 months	120	1.0–1.3	10
1 year	115	1.3–1.5	13
5 years	95	2.5–3.0	31
10 years	75	3.8–4.0	50
15 years	70	6.0	85

Source: Hazinski 1992

61

measured twelve hours after a meal and with the subject having rested for thirty minutes.) Food consumption, anxiety and anticipatory neuro-hormonal changes also change heart rate. Thus basal measurements for children are difficult to calculate. Heart rate reflects a decreasing BMR. In females this drops 23 per cent from the age of six years to sixteen years; their basal heart rate also reduces over this time by 20 per cent. Thus the growing child shows a decreasing BMR and a rise in heart stroke volume. Due to sinus node depolarisation, rate changes as the heart matures.

Exercise and cardiovascular function

Rate will rise as exercise increases because the volume will remain the same: the younger the child, the smaller the heart, the higher the rate at any given level of cardiac output or oxygen consumption. Pulse rates rise also on physical effort and in febrile conditions. Children's maximal heart rates are higher than adults, to a rate of approximately 200 beats per minute. Girls have similar maximal heart rates but significantly higher rates submaximally than similar aged boys. These differences appear at about the age of six years. Armstrong and Welsman (1997) suggest that this may be due to sex-related differences in autonomic cardiac regulation, which may also help to explain why boys have faster heart rate recovery rates following exercise.

Blood pressure and exercise

Resting blood pressure rises throughout childhood as the heart becomes bigger and stronger (see Table 4.4). Grossman (1991)

TABLE 4.3 Heart rates in childhood

Age	Awake	Asleep
Birth	100–180	80–160
3 months–2 years	80–150	70–120
2–10 years	70–110	60–100
10–adult	55–90	50–90

Source: Wong 1995

suggests that children of eight to ten years of age also demonstrate an ultradian rhythm, and that the development and maturity of the cardiovascular system and the underlying oscillator or pacemaker mechanisms may be a prerequisite to the achievement of adult blood pressure circadian rhythm, which would show a twenty-four-hour period.

Peripheral resistance factors such as sympathetic enervation of blood vessels, blood viscosity changes and local muscle response to metabolites are poorly researched at present. However, arterial blood vessels in children under one year have been found to contain fatty streaks regardless of sex, race, geography or hereditary factors, and these appear in the coronary arteries of children aged ten years. Studies have shown that 26 per cent of children in the two to twelve year age group have raised serum cholesterol (above the 5.2mmol/l recognised as maximum desirable). By the early teens most people have developed evidence of **atheroma** (Shuttleworth 1996). Whether lesions are reversible or precursors of fibrous plaques may be influenced by subsequent life events, but may have an effect on peripheral resistance at an early age and thus a rising blood pressure. A diet low in animal fats and junk food has been shown to reduce serum cholesterol in all age groups.

Children's response to exercise is thus related to their age, the type of exercise undertaken and the gradual effect of their lifestyle. There is normally a gradual rise in maximum systolic blood pressure as the child matures, and Armstrong and Welsman (1997) report some evidence that young people have a more favourable peripheral distribution of blood during exercise, which facilitates the transport of oxygen to the exercising muscles. Children have a slightly higher

TABLE 4.4 Blood pressure changes over childhood

Age	Male	Female
Newborn	70/55	65/55
5 years	95/56	94/56
10 years	100/62	102/62
15 years	115/65	111/67
Adult	121/70	112/60

mitochondrial density and oxidative enzyme availability than adults, and thus have an increased oxidative capacity of the muscle. Cardiac output of children may be much lower at the same oxygen uptake compared to adults; the child relies on a higher peripheral oxygen extraction.

At submaximal exercise levels increased oxygen extraction from the blood can compensate for the low cardiac output. At maximal levels this advantage is limited by the low haemoglobin content of the blood to transport oxygen to the tissues. Although there are no differences in early childhood, boys show an increasing haemoglobin concentration as they grow older when testosterone has an increasing effect on the growth spurt in their late teens. Girls, on the other hand, show an increase until menarche only, thus boys show superiority in endurance events.

Children's blood

The average blood volume in the full-term infant is 85ml/kg. Red cells are made in the red bone marrow which occupies most of the spongy spaces and medullary cavities of the skeleton in childhood. However, by puberty red marrow is replaced by yellow containing fat, and red cell production only remains in the upper shaft of the femur and humerus, vertebrae, sternum, ribs, innominate bones and scapulae. Reticulocytes are immature red cells that circulate in the blood and mature in two days. In the adult they make up 0.8 per cent of the blood cells. They are particularly evident when there has been blood loss as the marrow increases activity to boost the red cell count. For production the red marrow must have supplies of amino acids, iron, vitamins B12 and B6, and folic acid. Thus the child's diet is crucial to blood formation. Red marrow is stimulated to become active by erythopoietin, a hormone secreted from the kidney, and also by thyroxine, androgens and growth hormone. In emergencies the marrow can show a tenfold increase in productivity. In the three-month foetus, reticulocytes are 90 per cent of the circulation red blood cells, but drop to 2–7 per cent in the newborn and 0.5–1.5 per cent at three days of extra-uterine life.

Table 4.5 shows normal childhood haematology.

TABLE 4.5 Normal haematology in childhood

Age	Hb (g/dl)	MCV (fl)	WBC (10^9/l)	Plats
Birth	14.5–21.5	100–135	10–26	150–450
2 weeks	13.4–19.8	88–120	6–21	150–450
2 months	9.4–13.00	84–105	6–18	150–450
1 year	11.3–14.1	71–85	6–17.5	150–450
2–6 years	11.5–13.5	75–87	5–17	150–450
6–12 years	11.5–15.5	77–95	4.5–14.5	150–450
Male adult	13.0–16.0	78–95	4.5–13	150–450
Female adult	12.0–16.0	78–95	4.5–13	150–450

Source: Lissaeur and Clayden 1997

Note: Hb g/dl = haemoglobin (grams per decilitre). MCV = mean red cell volume, femto litres (1 femto litre = 10^{-12}g). WBC = white blood cell. Plats = platelets.

Common blood tests

Guthrie Test

This is to test for phenylalanine found in 1:7,000–10,000 live births. It is an autosomal recessive disorder. Excess of this chemical shows that the child's liver is not converting phenylalanine to tyrosine, an essential amino acid for tissue growth. Phenylketanuria (PKU) will lead to brain damage if undetected and not treated with an adjusted protein diet from birth. The child will usually be tested by heel prick on the sixth day of life after milk feeds have been established (Kelnar *et al.* 1993).

At the same time as the Guthrie Test, the child will be tested from the same heel prick sample for hypothyroidism, which is seen in 1:4,000 infants. This is a condition where, if not treated with replacement hormone which is essential for the development of brain and bones, cretinism develops.

In South Wales the blood test also screens for cystic fibrosis and other genetic disorders.

Routine diet supplement

Vitamin K

The newborn has two mechanisms for preventing bleeding; platelets and coagulation factors.

At birth platelets are above $100,000 \times 10^9/l$.

Coagulation factors are synthesised in the liver and depend on adequate vitamin K levels. These are low at birth and drop further in the first few days of life. Vitamin K is made in the gut by bacteria, but at birth the gut is sterile and only gradually becomes colonised during feeding, taking longer in breast-fed babies.

Vitamin K supplement is considered important for a healthy start to life; 0.5mg is given orally (or 0.1mg intramuscularly/intravenously) to all babies after the first feed, and two more doses of 0.5mg are given at seven days and six weeks.

Physiology knowledge in practice

Scenario

As the heart grows larger, the pulse rate will reduce. However, in any group of children of the same chronological age, these rates may differ. Explain what may affect pulse rate in the normal healthy child in relation to their weight and height.

Some pointers

Children have a relatively large surface area to mass ratio, which decreases with age. They become more stable in their density at three to four years of age. The calculation of body mass index (BMI) – kilograms divided by height in metres squared – must take consideration of body water and mineral content, physical activity, and the cultural/ethnic group. Also, boys show an increased muscle mass over the whole of childhood (see section on exercise in Chapter 3, and see Chapter 7 which deals with the digestive system). The 50th percentile range is shown in Table 4.6.

TABLE 4.6 Body mass index (BMI), 50th percentile range

Age in years	Male	Female
6	15.4	15.2
8	16.0	15.9
10	16.5	16.9
12	17.8	18.6
14	19.6	20.2
16	20.8	20.9

As the child grows bigger the heart will also grow and produce a larger stroke volume. Thus, at rest, the heart will beat slower to service the body tissues with oxygen and nutrients. Boys, who have more lean tissue – which has a higher metabolic rate – will also have larger hearts to service this need, thus their pulse rate at rest will be similar at a young age, slowing in the pubertal spurt when the testosterone surge is experienced. If the child is overweight the pulse will be higher, as the heart has to pump harder to circulate the blood around the adipose tissue, which will be well supplied with blood vessels, thus making the circulation longer than normal. In the underweight child the pulse may also be faster, perhaps due to the constant effect of adrenaline on the heart muscle if the child is anxious – a sympathetic nervous system effect. It may also be faster due to the high amount of circulating thyroxine, which also would boost all tissues to work faster and demand more oxygen supplies.

📖 *Extend your own knowledge*

Rowland *et al.* (1998) reported that the increasing involvement of children and adolescents in endurance sports competitions requires that professionals need a better understanding of cardiac response to exercise. They found that children did not develop increased left ventricular size as adults do, and that they could only improve their maximum oxygen uptake to 5–10 per cent with training. They suggested that there were other both qualitative and quantitative variables that needed to be explored. In a symposium report for the same journal, Gonzalez-Alonso (1998) found that dehydration caused by hyperthermia when exercising resulted in reduction of cardiac output, muscle blood flow, skin blood flow and blood pressure.

Q: How would the child's cardiovascular system be compromised if exercising for some time in the heat?

Chapter 5

The respiratory system

- Embryology of lung development
- Surfactant
- The lungs at birth
- Babies' breathing
- Apnoea
- Respiratory resuscitation
- The small child's breathing
- Changes in respiratory function at puberty
- Respiration changes during exercise
- Sleep and respiration changes
- Development of the ear

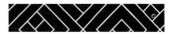

I N THE TERM infant there is a transition of breathing from episotic irregular, ineffectual movements to regular, rhythmic and effectual effort which is completed by the end of the first week of life. Respiratory rate, at seven days of age, will then show a response, increasing as does the adult response to hypoxaemia (low oxygen levels in the blood). Thus the main adaptation to air breathing has occurred at the end of week one. The respiratory system then grows and matures until eight years of age when the respiratory tree is completed. After this age environmental effects and changes in other body systems, especially those affected by sex hormones, may affect an individual child's respiratory function.

Embryology

Lung structure growth and development continues through the uterine and post-natal period, the embryonic stage commencing in the fourth gestational week on day twenty-two. The lung appears as a bud from the oesophagus below the pharyngeal pouches. Two branches, the bronchi, bud out on day twenty-six to twenty-eight, the right being larger than the left and orientated more vertically (Figure 5.1).

By the eighth week more branching has occurred from the bronchi, and hyaline cartilage is evident in their walls together with smooth muscle and capillaries. At seventeen weeks' gestation all structures are formed; the lung endoderm branching has occurred sixteen times to produce terminal bronchioles, but no gas exchange

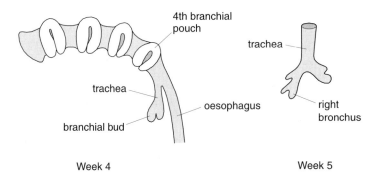

Week 4   Week 5

FIGURE 5.1   Lung buds at week four and bronchi at week five

is possible, thus the foetus would not be viable. From sixteen to twenty-five weeks terminal bronchioles become highly vascular, terminal sacs become thin-walled and some gas exchange is possible. Infants in this age range can survive, but they differ in their individual ability to do so. Babies under twenty-four weeks' gestation can be so fragile that they are at risk of permanent lung damage, but some grow up with healthy lungs due to advances in neonatal care. From twenty-four weeks' to birth the terminal sacs develop: about 20–70 million are formed in each lung by birth, and the total number in the adult will reach 300–400 million (Larsen 1993).

Foetal pulmonary resistance is very high; the lungs are filled with fluid so the alveoli are hypoxic. This ensures that pulmonary vaso-constriction occurs and thus only 8 per cent of the blood flows into the lung field, enough to nourish the developing pulmonary tissue (see Chapter 4 on the cardiovascular system). This hypoxia also leads to reduced breathing movements, as the reduction in move-ment reduces the overall oxygen demand of the foetus. Breathing is not important as the foetus receives its oxygen from the maternal circulation. At twenty weeks the bronchi and bronchioles' muscula-ture is complete. After this, muscle increases in the pulmonary arteries and the capillary beds develop round the terminal acinae. This leads to a reduction of pulmonary resistance in the third trimester of pregnancy. The baby shows frequent, shallow, irregular breathing movements in the second half of the pregnancy; its thorax will move in REM sleep for half to one-third of the time.

Surfactant

Surfactant is secreted from the type 2 pneumocytes in the alveoli walls. This counteracts surface tension forces and facilitates further terminal sac development

Surfactant is a lipid that is secreted on to the alveoli surface which prevents the sacs from collapsing on expiration by reducing surface tension on their internal surface. At twenty-two weeks' gestation surfactant is being secreted, with a surge in its production at thirty to thirty-five weeks and at birth (Kelnar *et al.* 1993). It flows up the trachea out of the mouth into the amniotic fluid; thus it can be tested at amniocentesis of the mother. Surfactant is a collection of fatty substances including much surface-active lecithins. Its production is reduced by intrapartum asphyxia from antepartum haemorrhage or maternal hypotension. Increase is promoted when the membranes have ruptured for more than twenty-four hours, placental infarction has occurred, in pre-eclampsia, or when hypertension with intra-uterine growth retardation is evident. Stress to the foetus causes gluco-corticoids to be released from the adrenal glands, and these stimulate surfactant release. Today, mothers in premature labour may be treated with betamethasone (a steroid) to protect their infants' lungs and small, premature babies may be given surfactant through their ventilator endotracheal tube with good effect.

The lungs at birth

The lungs of the foetus are filled with fluid until delivery. As the baby is squeezed through the vaginal canal the lungs are gradually squeezed of fluid, but the baby may need to be suctioned to remove residual mucus from the mouth and nose before it is swallowed. Residual fluid is then absorbed through the pulmonary capillaries and into the lymphatics. Mild cooling, light, sound, touch, odours and added gravity force, combined with the internal stimuli of reduced oxygen, acidity and rising carbon dioxide levels in the blood, to activate central and peripheral arterial chemo-receptors, stimulate the child to take its first breath of air. Now the lungs are taking in air they will not produce fluid. As the lungs expand, mechanical effects on the pulmonary arterioles allow them to dilate and blood flows to the lungs. The lungs then recoil away from the chest wall because of elastic fibres in the lung tissue, and the chest wall will spring out. Lung compliance then is determined by the amount of surfactant and lung elasticity.

The first few weeks

The infant is hypoxic at birth, and breathing shows a transitory bi-phasic structure. At first, ventilation responds to low oxygen but then drops to prehypoxic levels or below. This phenomenon adjusts to an adult response by day seven. The response may be due to mechanical factors involving the lungs and chest wall, delayed matu-ration of respiratory-related neurotransmitter systems in the brain and post-natal maturation of the peripheral arterial chemo-sensors system. In the first days of life the neonate also demonstrates intra-pulmonary shunting of blood due to the alveoli having some blocked and oedematous areas remaining. The poor perfusion of these sections of lung tissue results in a certain amount of hypox-aemia. Thus the oxygen pressures at day one may be 80mmHg and not peak for seven days. However, the carbon dioxide and blood acidity are normal over this time. In the preterm birth the infant will show diminished sensitivity to oxygen, as it still has the foetal response of elevated breathing movements reacting to rising carbon dioxide levels in the circulating blood.

In the first two to twelve weeks of extra-uterine life the muscles in the pulmonary arteries become thinner, dilate, lengthen and branch, which further reduces the resistance of the pulmonary vasculature and pressure of blood in the right side of the heart (Merenstein and Gardner 1998). However, the anatomy is still very reactive to hypoxia, acidosis, over-distension of the alveoli, and hypothermia. Over the next one to two months, the pulmonary vessels gradually function as in the adult, and throughout childhood the arteries develop muscle in those supplying the bronchi, bronchioles and alveoli. These changes, interestingly, may be delayed in children living at high altitude, those who are born prematurely and those with cardiac abnormalities.

Baby breathing

Babies up to four weeks are obligatory nose breathers, thus the risk to their breathing increases if they have colds or lie with their face in vomit or bedding. They do not adapt well to mouth breathing. They have small airways which will narrow further when swollen or blocked with secretions; thus they would have to work harder to breathe. Young babies who have difficulty with breathing have diffi-culty feeding and will soon lose weight (see Chapter 7 on the digestive system). Airway resistance in children is high due to this small diam-eter of their respiratory tree.

The patency of these upper airways is maintained by the active contraction of muscles in the pharynx and larynx. These muscles, if compromised when the neck is flexed or extended, will allow the airway to be compromised. The glottis is more cephalad in the baby than the five year old, the laryngeal reflexes more active and the epiglottis is longer. This will have importance if resuscitation is performed: the head position for artificial resuscitation aims to open the airway for re-breathing – the 'sniffing position' is thus recommended for small children under five years of age.

There is areolar tissue present below the vocal cords in young children which is not evident in the adult; this will swell and block the tracheal lumen if inflamed or traumatised. The narrowest part of the airway in the child is at this lower level of the cricoid cartilage, whereas in the adult it is higher, at the vocal cords which extend between the thyroid cartilage and the arytenoids. Vocal cords vibrate when air passes through the larynx; children have slender, short vocal cords and thus their voices tend to be high-pitched. At puberty, the larynx of a male will enlarge more than that of the female, and the vocal cords will become thicker and stronger and thus produce lower tones than the adult female.

The trachea is also very elastic and flexible in the young child. Babies have high tracheal **bifurcation** at the third thoracic vertebral level; thus they need their heads to be supported when handling and positioned with the jaw at right angles to the spine.

The respiratory tract is short and thus the risk of infective material entering is high. Small babies are susceptible to droplet spread of viruses and bacteria, e.g. colds and meningitis. The air sacs are not completed in number, and there is a smaller area for gas exchange. The round thoracic capacity, resulting from ribs lying horizontally, results in the diaphragm and abdomen being the primary means of ventilation. The diaphragm, enervated by the phrenic nerve, cannot contract as much or as effectively as in the older child because it is attached higher at the front of the chest and thus is relatively longer (Hazinski 1992).

Apnoea

This is a period of breathing absence lasting twenty seconds or more, or a shorter time if the child develops a bluish or pale colour or the heart rate drops. Many term babies have periods of rapid breathing alternating with periods of slow rate, or they may not breathe for periods up to fifteen seconds. This is normal if the colour and heart rate do not change considerably and the infant starts to breathe spontaneously. True apnoea is only common in young babies below thirty-two weeks. It can be prevented in these premature infants by minimal handling, keeping the child's temperature constant and lying the child in the prone position. Medically, they can be treated with caffeine, which quickly stimulates the central nervous controls of respiration.

Apnoea is caused by respiratory, central nervous system, metabolic and obstructive situations. The respiratory causes occur when the child is exhausted, has pneumonia or a pneumothorax, has aspirated some solid or fluid, or has had the vagus nerve stimulated in the pharynx. This last situation can be experienced when passing a feeding tube or over-suctioning a small child. Central causes are due to an immature respiratory control centre, which is most common, and when children have a seizure. Seizures can occur unexpectedly in **hyperpyrexia**, and are most often seen in children under five years of age whose temperature control mechanisms in the hypothalamus are also immature. Cerebral haemorrhage, cerebral birth trauma, **kernicterus** and meningitis are all rarer stimuli for apnoea, but breathing absence may be their first symptom. Metabolic effects of mineral deficiencies, low blood sugar and drug therapy can also quickly affect respiration rate, as well as congenital and secondary obstruction, such as the child's face being covered.

Respiratory resuscitation

This may be required as an emergency procedure if the child is choking (see Table 5.1). Procedures are based on Wong (1996), BMJ (1996) and Williams and Asquith (2000).

Assessment

- colour
- any vomit near face or clothing, etc.
- breathing effort
- sound of breathing effort
- return to breathing after bottom of feet flicked
- response to voice

TABLE 5.1 Resuscitation

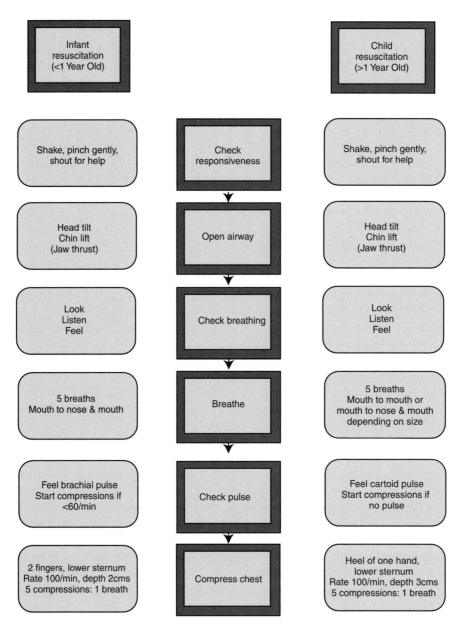

AFTER ONE MINUTE ACTIVATE
EMERGENCY MEDICAL SERVICES

Note: Computer work by Richard Hayward, Canterbury Christchurch University College. Adapted from the Resuscitation Guidelines 1997, produced by the Resuscitation Council.

Action

- note the time
- send for help

Infant

- if object clearly visible turn head to one side and remove object with one finger
- position infant face down with head lower than the chest
- give five quick blows between the shoulder blades
- give five chest thrusts with the infant in the supine position – position one finger below the nipple line

Child

- if object clearly visible turn head to one side and remove object with one finger
- place the child in the prone position with head lower than the chest
- give five quick blows between the shoulder blades
- give five chest thrusts
- position the older child in front of you and grasp round the waist
- give sharp abdominal thrust upwards
- repeat or lie child supine and continue abdominal thrusts

If the infant or child does not commence breathing:

- lie infant or child flat
- reposition the head to the 'sniffing position' or extend head if over eight years
- cover the nose and mouth with your mouth or pinch nose and cover mouth with yours in the older child
- attempt five slow rescue breaths of 1-1.5 secs and watch for the chest to rise
- if the chest does not rise, airway opening manoevres and rescue breaths should be repeated

If the child commences breathing:

- place in the recovery position in case of vomiting

- comfort the child
- document procedure

If the child does not respond:

- check pulse
- commence basic life support of a compression rate of 100/minute in infants and small children with a ratio of compression to ventilation of 5:1. In older children the ratio will be 15:2.

The small child's breathing

In a small child's respiratory effort the chest wall is compliant, as only the external intercostal muscles stabilise the chest wall. The diaphragm is more horizontal and there is lower rib retraction when the child lies supine. The greater the rib retraction the more the diaphragm will need to contract to generate tidal volume, thus this is a very inefficient way to breathe. Heat and water are transmitted to inspired air, thus children lose relatively more body heat and water from body tissues in breathing, so are more likely to develop mucus plugs when they have respiratory infections.

Airways increase in length and diameter after birth. Until three years the number of immature alveoli increase; after this the size only of the alveoli increases. Blood vessels are remodelled and increase in number while the new alveoli are forming. These terminal units increase in size and number until the age of eight years. Also, alveoli and bronchiole pathways for collateral ventilation (pores to allow trapped gas in obstructed airways to be absorbed) continue to develop until this age.

Changes at puberty

From five years to puberty the weight of the lungs increases threefold, vital capacity rises from 1,000 to 3,000cc, and total lung capacity improves from 1,400 to 4,500cc in the child on the 50 per cent percentile (see Chapter 10 for an explanation of percentile). Resting total lung volume increases as the lungs grow; this change is seen equally in boys and in girls. Respiratory frequency tends to be slightly higher in boys, perhaps due to their changing lean body mass as they approach puberty. Lean muscle tissue has a higher metabolic demand than fat. However, it must be remembered that the measurement of the peak expiratory flow depends on the child's effort and cooperation. Children using inhalers and monitors for their asthma must have age-related apparatus for their use, as effort will be related to their ability to coordinate breathing and blowing. Small children cannot conform due to immature central synchronisation controls or weak muscle function, and they often fear masks and restraint.

Maturation of the tissues is complete by eight years. From eight years to puberty increased air space occurs through enlargement of the alveoli and airways. Throughout childhood the volume of the lungs remains at a constant ratio to body mass. Lung capacity correlates best with the changing body height (Rowland 1996).

Ventilatory work, duration of inspiration and expiration are all influenced by resistance to flow in the airways and the elasticity – compliance – of the lung tissue. Resistance is created by friction of flow within both the lung and the upper airways. Compliance is determined by the elastic properties of the lung, connective tissues and the alveolar surface forces, as well as the chest wall. As the child grows and the airways enlarge, resistance reduces and respiration rate decreases. Compliance, which has improved most rapidly in the first two years, remains relatively high until five years. After this, compliance increases faster than resistance declines.

Table 5.2 details respiratory rates in children.

Respiration during exercise

Exercise increases demand for oxygen and production of carbon

TABLE 5.2 Respiratory rates in children

Age	Rate	Too high
Newborn	30–50	above 60
1 year	26–40	above 50
2 years	20–30	
4 years	20–30	above 40
6 years	20–26	
8 years	18–24	
10 years	18–24	
Adult	12–20	above 30

dioxide, which leads to increased alveolar ventilation, increased cardiac output and redistribution of blood to muscles. These three aspects are changing in the child as it grows and matures, and according to the lifestyle experienced. Up to a point the oxygen:carbon dioxide ratio remains the same. At a critical level anaerobic exercise takes place, where lactic acid production and bicarbonate buffering of hydrogen ions result in raised carbon dioxide for exhalation. Overall ventilation can increase twentyfold in exercise. Ventilation increases as the strength and rate of contraction of the respiratory muscles increases. Blood flow to the respiratory muscles increases by 5–12 per cent. In the lungs, perfusion of the pulmonary capillaries increases. There is a raised oxygen extraction by muscles as temperature rises and acidity of the blood falls. Also, oxygen unloading from the blood quickens.

Young people appear to have a more favourable peripheral distribution of blood during exercise, which facilitates the transport of oxygen to the exercising muscles. Children appear to have slightly more mitochondria and an elevated level of some oxidative enzymes in their body tissue cells when compared to adults, perhaps increasing the oxidative capacity of their muscles. However, they have significantly lower muscle cell glycogen stores than adults and they appear to be less able than adults to generate ATP (adenosine triphosphate) via glycogenolysis when performing strenuous (anaerobic) exercise for periods of ten to sixty seconds. Anaerobic performance increases with age; boys of eight years have only 70 per cent performance compared to boys of eleven years. Girls show a constant improvement with age; they peak in their teen years, but never achieve the performance of boys, whose anaerobic capacity increases further in puberty (Armstrong and Welsman 1997a).

Children hyperventilate during exercise, their patterns of ventilation changing as they grow. This is due to metabolic requirements being inversely related to age. Thus it may be due to age-related differences in lung size. It may also be due to neural controls, as the child has a lower set point for carbon dioxide, or to the size-related differences in the ventilation mechanisms. It may be due to their changing lung compliance and airway resistance. Children have changing lean:fat ratios as they move through childhood, and this will affect gas uptake; carbon dioxide may be stored in fat tissue. Children also have lower haemoglobin concentrations than adults; haemoglobin binds carbon dioxide and acts as a buffer to hydrogen ions. Children's oxygen uptake is at least as good as adults' but their movements are less efficient – they have a lower metabolic scope, smaller stores of muscle glycogen and immature temperature regulation systems. Thus, over long periods of aerobic activity, they are disadvantaged. Prolonged aerobic exercise during childhood must be approached with caution, especially if the environment conditions are adverse (Armstrong and Welsman 1997c).

During maximal exercise a five year old may have a minute volume of 35l, whereas an adult may reach 150l or more, minute volume being the depth (tidal volume) and rate of breathing. Children have shallower and more frequent rates but, related to body mass they have, interestingly, the same minute volume as adults. At any level of exercise smaller children breathe more to deliver a given amount of oxygen than do adolescents. Smaller children also appear to have a ventilatory drive more sensitive to carbon dioxide. As it is alveoli ventilation that drives gas exchange, and children have a smaller 'dead space' than adults, their alveoli ventilation is adequate for exercise (Armstrong and Welsman 1997c). Armstrong *et al.* (1994) showed that the sex difference between children's peak oxygen values in exercise, their aerobic fitness, can be attributed to habitual physical activity and haemoglobin concentration. Boys have been consistently shown to be more physically active than girls and show a greater percentage of lean body mass. Boys also show higher oxygen uptake even though their haemoglobin is similar to girls' in the pre-pubertal years.

At puberty, however, the differences are evident as boys develop a greater muscle mass and higher haemoglobin concentration under the effect of testosterone. Armstrong and Welsman (1997b) found that boys' maximum oxygen uptake increases by about 150 per cent over the age range eight to sixteen years, with girls demonstrating only an 80 per cent increase. They found that boys' values are about 13 per cent higher than girls at the age of ten years, with an increase to 37 per cent at sixteen years. However, Armstrong *et al.* (1994) showed that in twelve to sixteen year old males, body mass, age and height explained 74 per cent of the variance and serum testosterone did not significantly raise the scores.

In girls, Armstrong and Welsman (1997b) found that the accumulation of body fat in the pubertal years reduced their maximal oxygen uptake, whereas boys in the age range ten to sixteen years remained consistent to mass, age and height. Research continues on the effect of maturation on performance of respiratory function in older children, and how exercise can improve peripheral oxygen extraction in the developing cardiovascular system and muscles.

Sleep and breathing

We spend 30 per cent of our lives asleep. In non-Rapid Eye Movement (NREM) sleep, respiration is regular and ventilation reduces in relation to the reduced metabolic demand. This slowing of rate occurs as the child slips into stage two to four of the deep sleep state. The parasympathetic nerve supply dominates and the bronchi/bronchiole muscles relax and reduce lumen size. In Rapid Eye Movement (REM) sleep, respiration becomes irregular and the respiratory muscle activity is altered. Tonic intercostal muscle activity is partly abolished and rhythmic activity is reduced. Phasic diaphragm activity compensates. Arterial oxygen levels are reduced. There is a small decrease in ventilatory response to hypoxia, and loss of tonic and inspiratory phase is linked to relaxing of the **genioglossus muscle**. Tidal volume, the amount of air moved in one inspiration, reduces.

Small babies have longer REM sleep periods so are regularly seen to have irregular breathing. Any swelling of their upper airway will compromise their oxygen intake as the genioglossus muscle relaxes and the soft palate relaxes and the tongue falls back in the pharynx. A child in respiratory distress will become cyanotic (look pale), have nasal flaring, grunt and demonstrate retraction of tissue around the throat and chest. In the assessment of the child's respiratory system, the brain and central nervous system control, airway, chest wall, respiratory muscles and lung tissue all need to be considered.

Development of the ear

At birth the baby reacts to sound, of which the human voice is preferred; startle and blink reflexes occur at sudden noise. At one month the baby notices prolonged sounds such as a vacuum cleaner noise. At four months the baby will turn the head to voices and will quieten to familiar sounds; the baby will turn to noise from some distance by seven months and, at nine months, will listen attentively and show pleasure in babbling. At one year most babies will respond to familiar words.

The inner ear develops at each side of the hindbrain at four weeks' gestation, and the middle ear starts to develop from the first pharyngeal pouch at this time. The external ear then develops from the first and second branchial grooves and, until the twenty-eighth week of gestation, remains plugged with epithelial cells which will normally disperse before birth. Rubella virus contracted by the mother in the first trimester of pregnancy results in damage to the inner ear because the seventh week is a critical time for its formation. Debate within the profession on the danger of early sonar scanning of the pregnant woman in relation to ear damage in the foetus is interesting from this development point of view.

To examine the ear of a child, the appropriate size of equipment is necessary, together with an understanding of the anatomical changes that take place over childhood. The lobe of the infant ear should be moved down and back to straighten the upward-curving ear canal in order to visualise the tympanic membrane. In children over three years the canal curves downward and forward, thus the ear lobe needs to be gently pulled up and back.

Discussion about insertion of grommets surrounds the evidence that some children improve spontaneously from chronic infection of these tiny airways, yet others suffer hearing loss as great as 50 decibels (Moules and Ramsey 1998). Few children escape some symptoms of secretory otitis media (glue ear) in childhood, as upper respiratory infections of the throat, nose and ear are common at this time. The anatomy of the young child's upper respiratory tract is small and structures are relatively close together, thus infections such as the common cold causing inflammation of the lining mucosa in the nasal passages and pharynx will soon involve other associated structures in the ear. Strachan *et al.* (1989) indicated that passive smoking also puts children at risk because inhaled cigarette smoke impairs the mucociliary function in these nasopharyngeal tissues, causing an inflammatory exudate that blocks the tiny tubes.

When feeding the small child a semi-prone position is recommended, as it is less likely to cause reflux of milk into this narrow Eustachian tube (Figures 5.2 and 5.3) which joins the throat and middle ear.

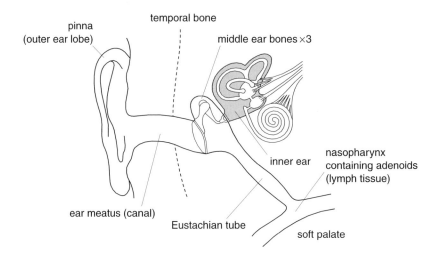

FIGURE 5.2 The Eustachian tube's position in the upper respiratory tract

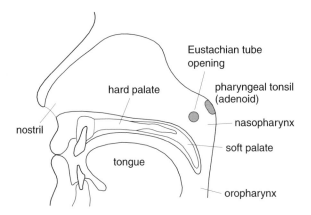

FIGURE 5.3 The Eustachian tube opening in the nasopharynx

Physiology knowledge in practice

Scenario

Children in infant schools can be seen to exercise in short, fast bursts. Many of them at the age of five years may be very tired at the end of the day in the first year of schooling. How is this activity pattern explained in relation to the young child's respiratory system?

Some pointers

Small children of five years do not have their complete respiratory airways formed; the alveoli are still developing, thus oxygen is not delivered to their tissues economically during activity.

They breathe shallowly and quickly to oxygenate their blood, but their intercostal muscles between the ribs are weak and have only limited glycogen stores, so respiratory effort is restricted until those energy stores are again available.

In a school day children in this age group are moving about constantly to satisfy their curiosity and to interact with their peers: many of them will be adapting from a slower, less stimulating environment.

Extend your own knowledge

Wibberley (1998), writing on young people's drug use, found that from 699 young people surveyed in the north of England, all accepted the use of recreational drugs as normal behaviour.

Q: In relation to changes in the respiratory control mechanisms when taking any recreational drug, what should health professionals understand when dealing with the emergency situation of a child who is addicted?

Chapter 6

The renal system

- Embryology of the urinary system
- The kidney and urine production at birth
- Fluid requirements in the first week
- Continence
- Bed wetting
- Water balance in children
- Urine
- Dehydration and rehydration

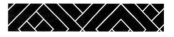

THE FUNCTION OF the renal system in childhood is critical to the healthy function of all body systems. Body water is the largest component of body tissues, comprising 70 per cent in the infant and decreasing to 60 per cent in the adult. In the child there is a higher amount of the water outside the cells in the interstitial spaces, and there is a higher turnover of water due to increased heat production and an immature kidney function to conserve water. Infants and young children also have a larger surface area:volume ratio to lose water and heat to the outside environment. They have a larger circulating blood volume per kilogram of body weight, but their overall volume is small, so loss of blood volume has a more devastating effect and quickly affects the vital body organs. Children take in water from their diet, normally controlled automatically by their sensation of thirst, a dry mouth and the hypothalamus thirst centre stimulus. They also produce water as a by-product of their high metabolic rate. They lose water mainly through their large skin surface, their relatively longer gut and their more rapid breathing.

Embryology

The urinary system develops from the **intermediate mesoderm** on either side of the dorsal body wall, which gives rise to three successive nephric structures of increasingly advanced design. The first are transitory, non-functional segmental nephrotomes in the cranial region which regress in the fourth week on day twenty-four to twenty-five. After this an elongated pair of mesonephroi appear in the thoracic and lumbar region either side of the vertebral column. These structures are functional, as they have complete nephrons and drain caudally via the Wolffian ducts to the urogenital sinus. By week five the ureteric buds (Figure 6.1) sprout from the Wolffian ducts and develop into definitive kidneys.

The bladder expands from the superior urogenic sinus and the inferior section gives rise to the urethra in both sexes. Ureters are then emplaced on the bladder wall. At week six germ cells migrating from the yolk sac induce the mesonephros to differentiate into Sertoli cells in the male and follicle cells in the female (see Chapter 8 on the reproductive system). At the same time a new Müllerian duct develops parallel to the mesonephric duct. In week six, when the Y chromosome exerts its effect, a development cascade then sees

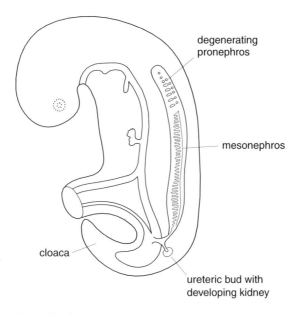

FIGURE 6.1 Kidney bud position

the forming of the male or female external genitalia and the kidneys ascending to their lumbar site in the abdomen, the right being lower than the left due to the presence of the liver.

By the tenth week, the foetal kidney is functional. Foetal urine is important, not to get rid of waste products from the blood as the placenta regulates fluid and electrolyte homeostasis, but to supplement the production of amniotic fluid. Foetal urine production may reach up to 200ml per day.

The kidney and urine production at birth

The neonate's kidneys weigh about 23g. This weight will double in six months and treble by the end of the first year (Sinclair 1991). The growth of the kidney depends on its work; if one kidney is removed the other will double in size.

At birth the loss of placenta flow, followed by a rapid increase in the infant's own renal blood flow, causes a high vascular resistance in the neonate kidney. This results in a temporary reduced renal blood flow and glomerulus filtration rate. The neonatal kidney has the normal million number of nephrons as in the adult, and their glomerulus capillaries' resistance reduces over the first few weeks of life, which allows increasing filtration ability.

The newborn kidney glomeruli capsules are formed of cuboid epithelium and are not fully replaced by thin pavement epithelium until after the first year of life. These small, immature glomeruli have short loops of Henle with distal convoluted tubules that are relatively resistant to aldosterone. This results in limited concentrating ability; maximum osmolarity approximately 800mosm/l compared to 1,200mosm/l in the two year old, and a reduced glomerulus filtration rate (GFR): 30ml/min/m^2 at birth, 100ml/min/m^2 at nine months, and reaching adult values at one year (Davenport 1996).

At birth, the renal cortex is underdeveloped and the juxtamedullary nephrons have higher blood flow than the cortical nephrons. This results in the neonate being better able to conserve sodium than excrete it. Difficulty in excretion of ammonium compounds and titrable acids impairs the ability of the kidney to correct acidosis, which occurs readily in very young babies. The regulation of the acid/base balance is quite well established, but there is limited ability to excrete hydrogen ions; thus babies will have limited response to a metabolic acidosis. Their serum pH averages slightly lower than normal at 7.3–7.35.

Interestingly, the maturation of the kidney relates to the load presented to it, and 95 per cent of babies will pass urine in the first twenty-four hours after birth. The new baby will pass 20–35ml of urine four times a day while intake is low as milk production establishes, but this soon rises to 100–200ml ten times a day by the tenth day of life. The urine that is produced has reduced maximal osmolality due to low urea excretion as growth, with its strong anabolic drive, assists the neonate kidney by reducing the excretion of sodium, water, phosphorus, hydrogen and nitrogen. Growth is thus sometimes referred to as the 'third kidney' (Halliday et al. 1989). There is no obligatory sodium requirement in the first twenty-four hours as glomerulus filtration rate is low and urine output small. Sodium needs remain low for three days because of isotonic loss of sodium and water (see section below on dehydration, p. 99). Table 6.1 presents a rough guide to electrolyte requirements.

For a few hours after birth there is a high urine volume with low concentration due to the immature sodium and water regulating system. After this, the water diuresis volume gradually decreases and

TABLE 6.1 A rough guide for electrolyte requirements

Sodium	2–4mmols/kg
Chloride	2–4mmols/kg
Potassium	1–3mmols/kg
Calcium	2–3mmols/kg
Magnesium	0.25
Phosphorus	2–3mmols/kg

Source: Halliday *et al.* 1989

Note: These levels are higher in the foetus but after birth fall until the parathyroid gland starts to function at three days.

concentrations rise. The newborn is then able to excrete amino acids and conserve sodium and glucose, but the ability to conserve and excrete free water remains immature so the baby is vulnerable to dehydration. Dehydration, hypotension and hypoxaemia all result in a marked fall in glomerulus filtration rate, so renal function becomes quickly compromised in the sick infant (Moules and Ramsay 1998).

Fluid requirements in the first week

Fluid requirements, ml/kg/24hrs, increase with weight. Turner *et al.* (1991) reported a survey of demand-fed infants and showed that they increased in their need for milk in the first week after birth (Table 6.2).

Milk intake appears to be highly individual, as is the timing, but a guide is often useful for the new mother. They should not over- or

TABLE 6.2 Fluid requirements, ml/kg/24 hours, in the first week after birth

Day	130–103ml
Day	250–130ml
Day	377–153ml
Day	480–170ml
Day	590–183ml

under-feed their babies from ignorance (see Chapter 7 on the digestive system). Young babies need to feed little and often, whereas older babies can take larger amounts of fluid less often. Fluid intake also has to be adjusted for ambient temperatures and the condition of the baby. The newborn infant has a surface area relatively two to three times that of the adult, thus a greater proportion of water will be lost through insensible routes.

Continence

In the infant, the bladder is an abdominal organ descending into the pelvis as more space becomes available. Thus the infant's ureter is relatively shorter than that of the older child and has no pelvic portion. The bladder is cigar-shaped and does not achieve its adult pyramid shape until about the sixth year. The posterior surface of the bladder is completely covered by the peritoneum.

The bladder is formed of four layers. The inner mucosa is folded into rugae and connected to the muscle layer by connective tissue. The bladder muscle, detrusor, is a sandwich of circular muscle between two layers of longitudinal muscle. The lower posterior wall is called the trigone, a triangular area where there are a large number of stretch receptors which respond to bladder filling. The base of the bladder neck joins to the urethra and here are the urinary sphincter mechanisms. At the neck of the bladder is a ring of smooth muscle, circular in the male and longitudinal in females, the internal sphincter. Below this, made of both smooth and striated muscle, lies the external sphincter. These are normally kept closed by the pelvic floor striated muscle (Colborn 1994) (Figure 6.2).

The ability to control bladder emptying is a process that is learnt usually in early childhood as a result of 'potty training'. A baby is incapable of exercising any control over this process, as bladder emptying is dependent on the action of the reflex arc (Figure 6.3). The bladder will voluntarily empty when stretched by a volume of 15ml, whereas the adult stimulus volume is 200ml. When the bladder fills it distends the trigone stretch receptors, and these in turn send impulses to the sacral area of the spine via the autonomic nervous system. Motor impulses from the spinal cord via the autonomic nervous system initiate relaxation of the internal sphincter and contraction of the detrusor muscle, leading to urine being expelled.

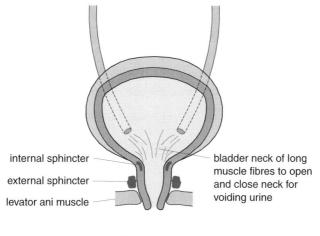

internal sphincter

external sphincter

levator ani muscle

bladder neck of long
muscle fibres to open
and close neck for
voiding urine

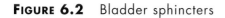
Renal system

FIGURE 6.2   Bladder sphincters

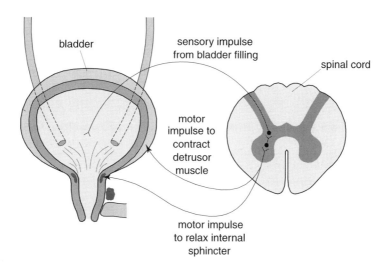

bladder

sensory impulse
from bladder filling

spinal cord

motor
impulse to
contract
detrusor
muscle

motor impulse
to relax internal
sphincter

FIGURE 6.3   The reflex arc for bladder emptying

Nervous system development is required for bladder control so
that the sensory impulses can travel via the spinal cord to the cerebral micturition control centre. Once awareness of the need to void
and of the social desirability to control micturition has developed,
together with the biological maturation of the nervous system and

93

the social development of the young, this becomes a controlled central nervous system activity which then blocks the reflex arc. Successful control usually starts at about two years of age when the child can voluntarily relax pelvic floor muscles in order to void. Consideration of the environment, timing and terminology in controlling micturition are all important to children attaining this control without embarrassment and stress.

Bed wetting – enuresis

This is a common problem in childhood, an alteration of neuromuscular function which is often benign and self-limiting. Rogers (1998) integrates several definitions of nocturnal enuresis to state that it is the involuntary passage of urine, during sleep, in a child aged five years or more, in the absence of any congenital or acquired defects of the nervous system. It is found in about 15 per cent of seven year olds and 1–2 per cent of teenagers. Wong (1997) has found that bladder control appears to be attained earlier in children in the UK and Sweden than children in the USA and those of Afro-Caribbean origin.

Bladder capacity, although differing widely among individual children, is generally greater in girls than in boys. Normal bladder capacity can be arrived at by taking the child's age and adding 2 in ounces and then multiplying by 30 (30ml = 1oz). For example, with a six year old child the calculation is 6 + 2 = 8oz $\times$ 30 = 240ml bladder capacity.

Children over the age of five years who wet the bed at night should be investigated in relation to tiredness, anxiety, infections and sleep pattern. Older children can become very embarrassed and restricted in their social life. Healthy bladders can be trained by good habits. Drinking adequately flushes out bacteria, and cleaning from front to back avoids contamination by rectal organisms. Children should also void as soon as they feel the urge to micturate, and sexually active girls should void soon after intercourse. Starting school, where toilets are shared and break times fixed, causes problems for some children, who will retain urine all day until they reach home.

Treatments include:

- behaviour modification
- psychological support for the child and the family
- reduction of fluids towards bedtime
- use of anticholinergic drugs which reduce uninhibited bladder contractions and vasopressin
- equipment such as alarms to wake children as they wet when asleep

Water balance

Water balance in children is quickly affected by environmental temperature and humidity; more so if they are physically active (see section on temperature control and exercise, Chapter 1, pp. 12–14). Table 6.3 shows daily fluid requirements for children of different ages.

Most babies lose weight in the first few days after birth. This drop is normally less than 10 per cent of the birth weight. Physiological weight loss is the result of fluid loss by evaporation from the skin,

TABLE 6.3 Daily fluid requirements for children of different ages

Age	Body wt (kg)	Total water (ml)/24hrs	Water (ml) /kg/24hrs
3 days	3.0	250–300	80–100
10 days	3.2	400–500	125–150
3 months	5.4	750–850	140–160
6 months	7.3	950–1100	130–155
9 months	8.6	1100–1250	125–145
1 year	9.5	1150–1300	120–135
2 years	11.8	1350–1500	115–125
4 years	16.2	1600–1800	100–110
6 years	20.0	1800–2000	90–100
10 years	28.7	2000–2500	70–85
14 years	45.0	2200–2700	50–60

Source: Metheny 1992

micturition, defecation and respiratory exchange. The first urine to be passed is colourless and odourless, with a specific gravity of 1.020 (Wong 1997).

The water content of an infant's body is 70–80 per cent, whereas that of an adult is 60 per cent. Of the newborn infant's water, 40 per cent is in the extracellular (EC) compartment compared to 20 per cent in the adult. As the baby grows, the ratio of extracellular to intracellular (IC) water decreases, due to cell growth in the tissues and the decreasing rate of growth of collagen relative to muscle tissue in the early months of life. Infants are vulnerable to water loss, however, because they ingest and excrete a relatively greater water volume each day. An infant may exchange half of his or her ECF daily, whereas the adult may only exchange one-sixth; proportionally the baby has less reserve of body fluid. The daily fluid exchange is relatively greater in infants, partly because their metabolic rate is twice that of adults per unit of body weight. Infants expend 100kcal/kg of body weight, whereas adults expend 40kcal/kg. Infants expel much body waste due to their high metabolic rate, so the kidneys need to form a large volume of fluid for this activity.

After the first year the total body water is about 64 per cent, at the end of the second year it is approaching adult levels, and by puberty the adult composition is attained, also showing the sex difference. Fat tissue contains little water; muscle tissue contains more, thus females have less body fluid than males and obese children have less than their lean peers.

The child's kidney becomes fully functional by the end of the second year. The small child has difficulty conserving water as it is needed to rid the body of wastes. The body surface and relative surface area of the gastrointestinal tract in childhood is relatively greater than in the adult, thus water loss from these surfaces is greater. Any increase or decrease in water and electrolytes has a greater effect. Metheny (1992) explains this as the child being a 'smaller vessel with a bigger spout'.

Urine

Collecting urine

Urine samples are often required of small children, and there are many ways to catch them. A mid-stream sample is the best, but difficult to obtain if the child is uncooperative. Older children can be washed with water round the perineal area and then instructed to allow some urine to pass into the toilet before they sample the urine into a sterile pot before completing their voiding. Another way is to attach a collecting plastic bag over the urethral opening, easier in boys than girls, or place a collection pad/cotton ball in the nappy/pants/knickers (Burke 1995). The carer can also be requested to catch a clean sample from a toddler who is left without a nappy until they void. This method is time-consuming but less traumatic for some children who have sore perineal areas.

Observing urine

Routine observation of the child's urine is helpful in detecting change in general health as well as for the laboratory test.

- Smell that is strongly ammoniacal may be the sign of infection; or if the child is taking medication the smell may reflect that of the oral preparation, e.g. antibiotic. Some foods also produce a characteristic smell in the urine, e.g. asparagus.
- Appearance should be straw coloured; if concentrated it will be a dark orange, and if diluted a pale lemon colour. Red urine may reflect the diet of the previous day, e.g. beetroot. Jaundiced babies will have a dark orange/brown urine due to the excretion of bile salts which should be excreted through the gut. Pink deposits from small babies are urates, not blood.
- Normal urinary output is about 1ml/kg/hr, increasing over childhood (see Table 6.4). Children who are dehydrated may not void for eighteen to twenty-four hours and still not have a distended bladder. However, some children are embarrassed to void in the presence of strangers or in strange environments; standing them or sitting them in an appropriate position will often get results. A child's bladder increases in size with age.

An approximate estimation of the volume from nappies or wet clothing is that 1ml = 1mg weight.

TABLE 6.4 Urine output by age

Age	ml
6 months–2 years	540–600
2–5 years	500–780
5–8 years	600–1200
8–14 years	1000–1500
14+	1500

Note: An approximate estimation of the volume from nappies or wet clothing is that 1ml = 1mg weight.

Testing urine

- Protein in the urine is normal in small amounts. This is due to the expulsion of dead cells that slough off from kidney nephrons, ureters and bladder lining. Levels will rise in the presence of infection as white cells are drawn to inflamed tissue.
- Glucose is not usually present unless the child is anxious, for example from injury or chronic stress, or has eaten a large amount of sugary foods.
- Ketones are commonly found in children who have not eaten recently, for example in the morning if they have not had breakfast or in the evening after a long day at school. Children who are feverish have a raised metabolic demand, as do children who are very active. Their bodies are breaking down their fat reserves to release energy as their glycogen stores are quickly used up if they do not eat. Release of ketones is the by-product of fat metabolism.
- The acidity of normal urine is 5.5, acidic. Small children often have a higher score as their urine is more alkaline due to their diet of milk and milk products. Children who have a high vegetable diet may also have an alkaline result.
- The specific gravity (SG) of urine is useful to detect dehydration, together with other observable signs such as small and infrequent volume passed. The specific gravity of water is 1,000, so the more solutes in the urine the higher the number will be. The child with a urine SG of 1,035 will need fluid input.

Dehydration

- Isotonic dehydration is when water and electrolytes are lost in equal amounts. The serum sodium remains at 130–150mEq/l, normal levels.
- Hypotonic dehydration (hyposmotic) is when the electrolytes are lost and the water concentration rises. The serum sodium is less than 130mEq/l.
- Hypertonic dehydration (hyperosmotic) is when there is water loss and retention of electrolytes. The serum sodium will be greater than 150mEq/l.

Infants are considered to be mildly dehydrated with 5 per cent water loss, moderately with 10 per cent and severely with 15 per cent. In the dehydrated older child the losses are lower at 3 per cent, 6 per cent and 9 per cent.

A child who is dehydrated will look flaccid, with sunken eyes that lack sparkle. A baby may present with a sunken fontanelle. It may be less inclined to eat, be less active and more irritable. It may have lost fluid through vomiting or diarrhoea. Weight may have been lost but blood pressure may be stable, although the pulse rate will rise as the circulating blood volume reduces. Tissue turgor begins to decrease when the child is 3–5 per cent dehydrated; this is best examined on the abdomen and thighs, but the obese child may seem to have a normal skin response, and malnourished children may have loss of turgor through their extreme thinness. A dry mouth can be ascertained by running the finger along the mucus membrane where the cheek and tongue meet; observation of the tongue will show it to be smaller than usual. The absence of tears and salivation are also useful signs. There is a significant loss from sweat if the body temperature attains 38.3°C or more or if the ambient temperature rises above 32.2°C. Body temperature will reduce as energy output decreases; however, dehydration often accompanies a fever as respirations rise and insensible loss occurs from the child's large surface area.

Oral rehydration

The solution recommended by the World Health Organisation contains sodium, potassium, chloride, base, glucose and water. Glucose is the preferred sugar because it facilitates the transport of sodium across the bowel wall. The usual recommendation when used to rehydrate children with diarrhoea is that the child takes this drink, volume calculated to the child's weight, each time there is a bowel action. It is also recommended for vomiting children if the solution is sipped frequently: a large volume taken quickly into an irritated gut will stimulate the vomit reflex. The electrolyte replacement is easily purchased in the UK in crystal form, and it can then be readily reconstituted with either cold or boiled tap water as required. Some of these products are flavoured to make them more palatable, as the salt taste can be unpleasant.

Over-hydration

Small babies cannot tolerate large intakes of free water because their **glomerular filtration** rate is low and they cannot dilute urine. Fluid retained in the extracellular spaces will produce dilutional hyponatraemia, water intoxication. As the extracellular sodium dilutes, water moves into the cells and cerebral and pulmonary oedema develops. This condition can occur if babies are fed dilute formula milk, take in excess water from bathing and are given inappropriate glucose solutions for thirst (Metheny 1992).

Replacement of body electrolytes by diet

- When children vomit they lose the gastric acid which causes a **metabolic alkalosis**. The kidney attempts to conserve hydrogen ions from the collecting tubules to correct this disturbance, and in the process losses to urine of potassium occur. If the child can eat, bananas, dates and raisins are high in potassium and can be used more safely that medications to replace it.
- Professional athletes can be seen to use both electrolyte fluids and potassium-rich foods such as bananas to compensate for

potassium loss. In excessive sweating sodium is lost through the skin, so the body conserves sodium and expels potassium via the kidney.

Physiology knowledge in practice

Scenario

Children are bringing crisps and cans of fizzy drink to school for mid-morning break, and many are having the same menu for lunch. How do these two items affect the child's renal system and result in their constant desire to buy more cans of drink?

Some pointers

- Crisps contain salt, a sodium load for the bloodstream. This will increase the solute of the plasma and its osmotic pull, thus water will be drawn from the interstitial spaces (ICS) into the blood. This, in turn, will draw water from the cells.
- The more 'concentrated' blood will stimulate the osmoreceptors in the hypothalamus, which will detect a rise in **osmolality** in the extracellular fluid and will initiate a neural circuit that results in the conscious sensation of thirst.
- In the kidney, the rise in ADH (anti-diuretic hormone) secretion from the posterior pituitary, mediated via the osmoreceptors, leads to increased water reabsorption at the nephron distal tubule. Small volumes of urine will be voided.
- As more and more fluid is reabsorbed from the ICS and ingested via the gut, it dilutes the sodium in the blood and is eventually flushed from the body and urine output increases.
- The intake of a very sweet drink raises the blood osmolality further and increases rather than decreases dehydration and thirst (Bridle 1994).

Extend your own knowledge

Bath and Morton (1996) found that in a sample of twenty-six children in the UK who continued to wet the bed at night, all had small nocturnal bladder capacity. They suggested that behavioural techniques should be continued and that practitioners should not resort to medications. Goin (1998), in a review of practice in the USA of enuresis management, found that five million children suffered with the problem and supported Bath and Morton's findings that behavioural techniques were superior of all the approaches in addressing this problem. He asked why hypnosis was not more commonly used.

Q: What is the psychophysiological explanation for the positive results found by these two researchers in the treatment of enuresis with behavioural techniques?

Chapter 7

The digestive system

- Embryology of the gut
- The baby's mouth and sucking
- Reflexes of the mouth and throat
- Baby feeding
- The developing gut
- Weaning
- Failure to thrive
- Calorie needs
- Teeth
- Liver maturation
- Physiological jaundice
- Bowels and stools

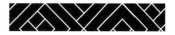

THE IMMEDIATE AIM of feeding children is a happy growing child, and if the child is happy and growing the carer's method is probably a good one, even if it is unusual (MacKeith and Wood 1971). Thus a discussion of nutrition must remain embedded in all aspects of children's lives, which include their developing anatomy and physiology.

Malnutrition has effects on the physical development of children and can include impaired gastrointestinal function, growth failure, puberty delay, impaired brain growth function in infants, developmental delay, immune deficiency with increased susceptibility to infections, respiratory dysfunction, muscle wasting and altered mood and behaviours.

Embryology

In the embryo, the primitive digestive tract is a tube consisting of three parts: the foregut, the midgut and the hindgut which develop from the yolk sac. The foregut gives rise to the pharynx, lower respiratory system, oesophagus, stomach, first and second sections of the duodenum, liver, pancreas and biliary apparatus. The midgut ranges from the duodenum to the transverse colon and the hindgut develops into the rest of the gut to the anus. Due to herniation of the midgut into the umbilical sac at week six to ten of foetal life, the mesentary is fixed at the top in the left upper quadrant of the abdominal cavity by the ligament of Treitz and at the bottom in the right iliac fossa.

These anatomical combinations explain how some babies are born with strange anomalies such as the oesophagus and trachea joined together, and abdominal contents which have grown outside the skin covering of the abdomen rather than inside it.

The mouth

When a baby is born it is suddenly separated from its source of nutrients in the maternal circulation; thus the neonate may lose 5–10 per cent of its body weight due to this shock of birth.

At birth the infant's lips are well adapted to closing round a nipple to feed. They are usually parted and show 'sucking blisters' or *pars villosa*. These keep the seal when the baby sucks. At rest, the back of the mouth is firmly closed with the tongue against the palate if not swallowing. In feeding, the baby draws the nipple far back into the mouth, then squeezes milk by elevating the dorsum of the tongue from the front to the back against the hard palate. The gums then open, the tongue slides forward and the system refills with milk. This stripping and swallowing cycle then repeats (see Figures 7.1 and 7.2). There is usually a rhythm of one breath to one or two swallows. The efficiency of this system increases from week forty of gestation.

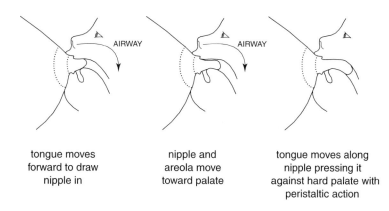

tongue moves forward to draw nipple in

nipple and areola move toward palate

tongue moves along nipple pressing it against hard palate with peristaltic action

FIGURE 7.1   Sucking from the breast

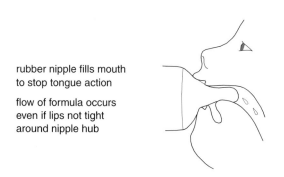

rubber nipple fills mouth to stop tongue action

flow of formula occurs even if lips not tight around nipple hub

FIGURE 7.2   Sucking from the bottle

Very premature infants do not have this ability and may have to be fed by tube until they are mature enough, and all babies with blocked noses will have this rhythm broken and may not feed adequately. New babies appear to accept both breast and bottle nipple quite readily, but as the skill is perfected nipple preference becomes evident. Breast feeding may become more difficult if the baby is fed complementary or supplementary infant formula milk from a bottle. Breast milk is provided on a supply and demand basis, i.e. if the baby is prevented from 'fixing on' to the breast, the 'let down' reflex is not stimulated and this can result in a reduction of breast milk production for the next feed. The teat of the breast and the bottle are different in shape and texture; small babies are expert at the one they prefer. Many mothers have a battle to wean their child off the breast and try many shapes of teat to pacify their offspring. Yet others find that if the bottle is the chosen method of feeding due to sore nipples or exhaustion from the baby's constant snacking, the baby will not work to gain nourishment from the breast, having found it easier to gain food from the artificial source.

The pharyngeal-oesophageal swallow is a primitive function but the child's mouth quickly learns discriminative and motor skills. In the first few months the suck and swallow will progress to manipulation of more solid food without gagging. Only small amounts of saliva containing the enzyme amylase are produced by the salivary glands in the neonate with little enzyme function; these develop full function by the age of two years. All babies have taste and smell present at birth, and all young babies can soon learn to like sweet tastes distinguished by the taste buds at the tongue tip, soft palate and inside of the cheek. If oral medications are sweetened children are usually happy to cooperate if a small amount is introduced at the front of the mouth. Breast milk is sweeter than artificial feeds, and breast-fed babies appear to enjoy fruits as their first foods. The ability to suck semi-solid food, bite and chew appears at five to six months and lumpy food can be tolerated at the six to seven month 'sensitive period' for this motor ability. However, many children will gag or spit out lumps for many months.

Physical assessment of the mouth

- intact high-arched palate

- uvula in the midline
- frenulum of the tongue
- frenum of the upper lip
- sucking reflex which is strong and coordinated
- gag reflex
- extrusion reflex
- absent or minimal salivation
- vigorous cry

Reflexes of the mouth and throat

- sucking
- gag – stimulation of the posterior pharynx
- rooting – touching cheek stimulates movement towards touch (goes four to twelve months)
- extrusion – if tongue is touched or depressed the response is to force it out of mouth (goes at four months)
- yawn – response to lack of oxygen
- cough – response to irritation of the mucosa of the larynx, trachea, bronchii

(Wong 1996)

The stomach

Prior to birth the gastrointestinal tract is filled with fluid and the remnants of the developing bowel lumen as it grows and sheds the lining. By five months of pregnancy the foetus is swallowing small amounts of liquor amnii, lanugo hair, **desquamated epithelium** and bile excreted from the liver. This is called the meconium. At the first few breaths after birth the infant swallows air; in three hours the whole gut contains gas.

As the child feeds so gas is taken in. A 3.5kg baby will take in 100ml of milk in fifteen minutes and the same volume of air. The best position to 'burp' a baby is to hold it sitting supported at the back and neck so as to allow the gas to bubble up a straight oesophagus. Patting a baby on the back may be comforting for the carer to have a physical communication, but gas will rise to the top of a bag of fluid, so if the stomach is positioned with the cardiac sphincter of the stomach upright the baby will bring the wind up to the mouth. 'Windy' babies are often more comfortable propped up for an hour, carried upright looking over the carer's shoulder, or placed on their abdomen over a carer's lap after a feed, so that wind can be expelled, before being put to sleep flat (supine) on their backs. At present, with the advice to lie babies only on their backs to avoid cot deaths from suffocation, many mothers are reluctant to use the face-down position.

The position and shape of the stomach is high in the abdomen and is orientated transversely rather than vertically as in the older (seven to ten years) child. The capacity of the stomach changes with age (see Table 7.1).

At birth the abdomen and thorax are of equal circumference. All muscles in the body are poorly developed, thus the abdomen will appear prominent. Muscle development also affects the lower oesophagus tone, an important barrier to preventing the reflux of stomach contents.

Infants breathe using abdominal movement, and this pot-bellied appearance will persist sometimes until eleven years of age when the abdominal muscles strengthen and the vertebral curves develop. In observing small children's respiration or monitoring their respiration rate, the abdominal movement is used together with chest compliance, tracheal tug and nasal flare. Apnoea alarms are fixed to the abdomen skin surface in children under the age of six months to monitor those with respiratory risk.

TABLE 7.1 Stomach capacities by age (in mls)

Newborn	10–20
1 week	30–90
2–3 weeks	75–100
1 month	90–150
3 months	150–200
1 year	210–360
2 years	500
10 years	750–900
16 years	1500
Adult	2000–3000

Source: Moules and Ramsay 1998

Swallowing is an autonomic reflex for the first three months of life until the striated muscles in the throat establish cerebral connections. Emptying time for the newborn's stomach is two and a half to three hours (the five year old's is three to six hours). By six months the baby is capable of swallowing, holding food in the mouth or spitting it out. The pelvic bones are still relatively small so the pelvic viscera remain placed higher than in older children. Thus this raised intra-abdominal pressure, vertical lie of the stomach altering the angle of entry of the oesophagus into the fundus and rapid peristalsis, predisposes the baby under six months to posset easily after feeds, especially if excess air has been taken while crying or sucking. The functional immaturity of the lower oesophagus 'sphincter' (Figure 7.3) also leads to episodes of inappropriate relaxation, and the short intra-abdominal length of this tube contributes to the baby being able to readily bring back feed.

Hydrochloric acid present at birth falls too low to permit much peptic acid digestion of protein in the stomach. The pH is nearly neutral (pH7) at birth due to swallowing of the alkaline amniotic fluid, but in the first eight hours of life gastric secretion does commence. The stomach, however, is more important for coagulating the casein of milk and controlling its passage to the small intestine. Curd (casein) may stay in the stomach and be gradually broken down in the pyloric antrum over the next twenty-four hours, whereas

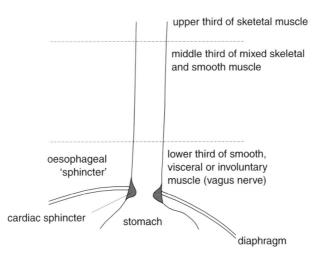

FIGURE 7.3   The oesophagus sphincter

the whey will move through to the duodenum within an hour. Acid secretion reaches adult levels at about ten years, when children become less likely to develop gastroenteritis as the acid will kill bacteria from oral intake more completely.

Colostrum, a clear fluid produced by the mother soon after birth, is high in globulins, especially IgA, which are also received by the infant via the placenta. It is high in a protein that is easy for the baby to digest. After one or two days milk supply is evident and within a week the supply is established.

Sugars in human milk contain e-fructose, a growth factor for lactobacillus bifidus, which is not found in cow's milk. This bacterium raises gut acidity and thus inhibits e.coli bacterial growth in the bowel. Breast milk is not sterile and contains some bacteria; thus it must be boiled if stored for longer than twenty-four hours. HIV passed from the mother in breast milk should not be used or donated to others.

The gut

Digestion is the process where food is broken down in the gut to simple substances that can be absorbed into the blood and lymph. Food must be appropriate to the stage of maturation of the entire gastrointestinal tract. Most biochemical and physiological functions are present at birth; secretory cells are functional but mature in efficiency with age (Moules and Ramsay 1998). The pancreatic secretions are sufficiently mature for a milk diet, and lactose (milk sugar) can be digested from forty weeks' gestation. This lactase enzyme activity is high in the small intestine at birth, but declines during infancy and is lost by adult life in many individuals. Amylase, a pancreatic enzyme that breaks down carbohydrates, and enterokinase, which is secreted from the ileum mucosa to activate trypsin for the breakdown of protein to peptides, are also present in the neonate gut. In the first three months pancreatic juice contains only a little lipase, which limits the baby's capacity to convert fat into fatty acids and glycerol. Specific long-chain polyunsaturated fatty acids (LCPs) are present in breast milk to feed the large developing brain; thus nature has matched the milk supply to the young animal's physiology.

First foods of ground rice and fruits are thus more easily digested.

It is interesting that in the first six months only small amounts of pancreatic amylase are produced to digest complex carbohydrates: could it be suggested that this may be a reason for colic at this time? If foods are too complex, the lack of digestive enzymes allows material to pass undigested to the colon, where the rise in osmotic pressure will draw water from the interstitial spaces and lead to increased peristalsis and loose stools.

As children move from food which is bland, simple and of a smooth consistency to one that is taken from the family choice, bowel irregularity is common. Toddler diarrhoea, however, is self-limiting, and most children appear to thrive throughout this period of faddy feeding and constant, smelly, loose stools. The digestive system only gradually develops the ability to digest more solid foods over the first two years and there may be maturational delay of gut motility. As acid levels in the stomach rise, so protein digestion improves due to the activation by acid of the stomach enzyme peptin.

Weaning

Weaning programmes which are recommended from four months incorporate the need to increase the consistency and texture of solid foods at this age (Gilbert 1998). However, some babies are reluctant to try at the first attempt and will gag; they may prefer smooth texture for a few more weeks. Saliva, at first, contains little starch digesting enzyme (salivary amylase) but at three months it increases, and cereals can be digested and biscuits sucked soft enough to eat at six months. Rice is recommended as a first cereal because of the possibility that an allergy to gluten may occur in some children (1:2,000). Wheat, oats, rye and barley contain gluten but rice and maize do not. Choking on large lumps is still a danger at this age. Pipped, seeded or skinny fruits, nuts or highly spiced foods need a mature digestive system, good teeth and the ability to avoid accidental inhalation. After six months a mix of foods is necessary to provide sufficient energy, trace elements (especially iron) and vitamins. Vitamin C is needed daily as it is not stored in the body. Sodium levels will be excessive if unmodified cow's milk is given as the only milk source from birth; cow's milk protein is also difficult for the child under one year to digest and, if given as the main 'food', is thought to be one of the common causes of iron deficiency anaemia in this age group. In fact, salty foods should be restricted for the first few years of life as sodium intake has been implicated in the onset of hypertension in adulthood. Bags of crisps and other salty snacks are not recommended as a frequent 'filler'. At this age 7 per cent of total energy from food is needed for actual growth, as opposed to energy for maintenance and activity. 'Nursery food' that is dense in calories is preferred, offered at routine mealtimes so that snacking habits are not encouraged in these capricious eaters (DOH 1994).

Failure to thrive

Children who fail to thrive from feeding problems can be classified under 'too little in', 'failure to utilise nutrients' and 'too much out'.

Too little in

- physical feeding difficulties
- excess vomiting
- anorexia
- ignorance of feeding requirements or poverty – fizzy sweet drinks between meals dull the appetite

Failure to utilise nutrients

- genetic conditions – cystic fibrosis
- congenital diseases – gluten allergy
- cow's milk allergy
- severe infestations – worms

Too much out

- infections – e.g. rotavirus, e.coli and campylobacter
- 'toddler diarrhoea' – common when the child moves from a pappy, liquid diet to a more mixed diet of adult foods (Kerrigan 1996)
- chronic conditions, e.g. diabetes

Calorie needs as basic metabolic rate (BMR) changes

Changes in height lead to changes in shape and basic metabolic rate. As surface area reduces to body mass and size increases, so calorie needs per kilogram reduce. Basic metabolic rate, when the individual is at rest, is where energy released from food meets the needs of the heart, lungs, nervous system and kidneys, and excess is lost as heat through the skin. Surface area in square metres is calculated from the height and weight of the individual. However, age, sex, menstruation, eating/starving, exercise, fever and thyroid function must all be considered when assessing rate of calorie use. Table 7.2 shows estimated average requirements for dietary energy.

The calorie needs of the preschool child (one to five years) are not as high as of the infant. However, they need a gradual change of eating pattern to adult equivalent at five years. Small children need frequent varied meals and snacks of foods high in nutritional value. Sweet and salty food needs to be restricted as snacks, especially for the faddy eaters.

Cereal and milk products contribute the most to energy, supplying protein, iron, calcium, zinc, vitamin A, vitamin B and riboflavin. Fruit drinks contribute to vitamin C intake. Thus a good breakfast of cereals, toast and milk is important for children of the junior school age group.

The main source of energy for the adolescent appears to be bread, chips, milk, biscuits, meat products, cake and puddings. 'Fast foods', high in fat, salt and sugar, and which can be eaten at random,

TABLE 7.2 Estimated average requirements for dietary energy, kcal/day and protein g/kg/day

	Dietary energy kcal/day	*Protein g/kg/day*
0–6 months	115	2.2
6–12 months	95	2.0
1–3 years	95	1.8
4–6 years	90	1.5
7–10 years	75	1.2
11–14 years	65/55	1.0
15–18 years	60/40	0.8

Source: DOH 1991

appeal to adolescent culture. 'Food groups' – meat, milk, fruit and vegetables, cereals and fats – may help these older children to choose their diet more sensibly.

Table 7.3 shows expected weight gains for developing children.

Teeth

Teeth may be present in the newborn but generally they start to erupt at about six to eight months; the lower two central incisors are usually first. Some babies do not commence teething until twelve months, although they have dribbled and chewed their fists for weeks. Teething does lead to an increase in salivation and babies may have loose stools, ammoniacal nappy rash, a raised temperature and cough (MacKeith and Wood 1971). But there is controversy on this point. There is also controversy on symptoms experienced by some babies, as some have no problems at this time and others are unhappy for days. The complete set of deciduous teeth numbers

TABLE 7.3 Expected weight gains for children in the UK – weight and age to show change in relation to height over the early years

Age	Weight	Height
Infant–6 months	Weekly gain 140–200g. Birth weight doubles by end of first 4–7 months	Monthly gain 2.5cm
6–12 months	Weekly gain 85–140g. Birth weight triples by end of year one	Monthly gain 1.25cm. Birth length increases by 50% end of year one
Toddlers	Birth weight triples by 14–17 months. Birth weight quadruples by 2.5 years. Yearly gain 2–3kg	Height at 2 years approx. 50% of eventual adult height. Gain in year 2: 12cm. Gain in year 3: 6–8cm
Preschool age	Yearly gain 2–3kg	Yearly gain 5–7.5cm
Junior school age	Yearly gain 2–3kg	Yearly gain 5cm. Birth length triples by 13 years
10–14 years (females)	7–25kg	5–25cm. 95% of mature height by onset of menarche
10–14 years (males)	7–30kg	10–30cm. 95% of mature height by 15 years

Source: Campbell and Glasper 1995

twenty, and is achieved by thirty months; they should be carefully guarded. Sugary drinks in bottles will rot the thin enamel: lost teeth at this time may disrupt the even eruption of the permanent set later. In the first year of life the baby has no molar teeth so cannot chew thoroughly, and the deciduous teeth are blunt.

At six to eight years the deciduous teeth will begin to be lost in the same order they were grown, but the full set of adult teeth may not arrive until adolescence. Today there are many adults without the full set of thirty-two teeth which include the 'wisdom' teeth molars. This may be an inherited characteristic or the effect of environmental changes over generations.

Liver maturation

At birth 40 per cent of the peritoneal cavity is occupied by the liver which displaces the bowel. The hepatic flexure of the colon moves to lie at a lower level than the splenic flexure. The transverse colon moves higher and the small bowel lies centrally in the abdomen.

Physiological jaundice

The neonatal liver is functionally immature. It lacks enough of the enzyme required in the production of bilirubin, which is formed from the oxidation of the *haem* of haemoglobin. This enzyme system develops, usually, within two weeks of birth. Thus jaundice frequently occurs in the first two weeks of life. Jaundice occurs when there is a rise of bilirubin in the blood. Normal levels are below 1.5mg/ml and jaundice is detected if the levels rise above 3mg/ml. It can be seen in the sclera, soft palate and skin, as the bilirubin is retained in the blood plasma and excreted via the kidney rather than through the liver into the gut. Normally the liver will bind bilirubin to albumin in the plasma and add a sugar molucule to form conjugated bilirubin, which is water soluble and excreted in the bile via the gut. If this process does not happen the bilirubin is not conjugated to sugar and is lipid soluble, which is why it permeates into the body tissues. Physiological jaundice, present in 15 per cent of healthy breast-fed babies, is caused by this immature hepatic function and a rise in the bilirubin load from red blood cells which haemolyse rapidly after twenty-four hours of birth. Red cell life span of the newborn is seventy days as compared to 120 days for adults, therefore breakdown occurs more frequently in the young baby. This type of jaundice is made more severe if the baby becomes dehydrated due to inadequate feeding. The bilirubin will make the child sleepy and reluctant to feed and thus be at risk of becoming dehydrated. The bilirubin will also be reabsorbed from the gut rather than expelled; bile in the gut will make the stools dark green and loose, increasing the dehydrated state.

Bowels

The rectum is a straight muscular tube with a simple columnar epithelium lining. This mucus membrane is thick but loosly connected to the muscle coat beneath. This favours prolapse, especially in children. The muscular trunk is relatively thick compared to the rest of the digestive tract. The anal canal is the last centimetre that ends in the anus. Here the smooth muscle layer is even thicker than the rectum and forms the internal anal sphincter (Figure 7.4) at the superior end of the canal. At the inferior end lies the external anal sphincter composed of skeletal muscle (Figure 7.4). The external sphincter is a flat sheet of muscle, elliptical in shape and adherent to the skin round the anus. It is enervated from the fourth sacral vertebra and is normally in tonic contraction because it has no antagonistic muscle. Thus it keeps the anal orifice closed and can be tightened at will. Any medications administered to children rectally must be introduced gently to overcome this tight control, as children will tense with anxiety. Once inserted, however, solid and liquid preparations will be retained well.

Waste products move through by stimulus originating in the stomach after a meal. This peristaltic contraction moves through the gut and commonly occurs fifteen minutes after breakfast. Distension of the rectal wall by faeces stimulates the defecation reflex of the internal sphincter. This reflex persists for only a few minutes before it is extinguished. Good training to respond to this reflex will ensure that good bowel habits are formed and comfortable stools passed. **Parasympathetic reflexes** then produce strong contractions. Nerve signals from the internal sphincter move to the sacral region, where nerves are stimulated to reinforce peristalsis in

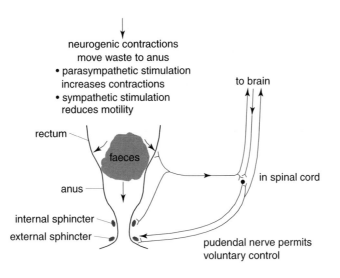

neurogenic contractions
move waste to anus
• parasympathetic stimulation
  increases contractions
• sympathetic stimulation
  reduces motility

to brain

rectum

faeces

in spinal cord

anus

internal sphincter

external sphincter

pudendal nerve permits
voluntary control

FIGURE 7.4 Internal and external anal sphincters

the colon and the internal sphincter relaxes to allow passage of the stool out of the anus. If children have to wait to pass a stool they will lose the urge to push. They will, then, retain the faeces in the large intestine where water will be extracted and a harder, more constipated stool formed.

In the small baby a stool is passed in relation to eating; also the toddler will have a regular 'poo' after breakfast and some mothers will recognise this fact and 'potty train' their offspring from birth. However, this is a reflex action for more than two years rather than a conscious decision by the child! Small children cannot control their bowel until their nervous system has matured to allow them central nervous system control. Their stool is passed simply when the rectum is full.

The external sphincter, under conscious cerebral control, will eventually prevent or allow defecation as appropriate. This is often accompanied by voluntary movements to help expulsion, such as taking a deep breath, closing the larynx and contracting the abdominal muscles. The pressure in the abdominal cavity then rises and forces the faeces out. Again, some mothers recognise this moment and sit the child on the potty successfully and reward the behaviour positively.

This is the start of potty training. However, many children see this as a game and do not understand, while others will resist the urge due to attention-seeking behaviour or anxiety, and become more and more constipated as the urge fades quickly. At twenty-four to thirty months children may have reached readiness for daytime control of the bowel; they will then exhibit the usual range of motion frequency in the general population. On starting school, where shared toilets may be embarrassing for some children, or where anxiety about punishment is a problem for others, children of five years and above may regress temporarily in this ability. Consistent faecal soiling, however, is abnormal over the age of four years (Lissauer and Clayden 1997).

Babies' stools

The stools of the newborn (meconium) are odourless, dark green and have a smooth, paste-like appearance. They are composed of digestive juices, desquamated cells and amniotic fluid which is passed in the first two days of life. The transitional stools are slightly porridge-like, yellow in colour and have a more sour smell. These may be passed several times a day if the baby is breast fed. Water, casein, fat, fatty acids, mineral salts and live and dead bacteria are present in faeces. Enzymes such as proteases, lipases and urases will interact with urine urea to increase pH (acidity). Breast-fed babies' stools have a lower pH than babies fed on infant formula milk, due to the fermentative gut flora, b.acidophilus, which produces neutral and acid metabolic waste products. When the pH drops, the faecal enzymes become less active and thus these breast-fed babies usually have less nappy rash. Bottle-fed babies have scanty b.acidophilus and pass firmer, paler stools which can smell foul due to fatty curd which is often present with some mucus. Excess protein will promote a stool that is firm and shows evidence of solid particles of casein. Excess sugar in the diet will act as a mild aperient because sugar increases the osmotic pull of water into the gut. Underfed bottle-fed babies will often pass small constipated stools, as will babies who are well fed but dehydrated; they may, alternatively, become more like meconium and be passed frequently in small amounts.

Physiology knowledge in practice

Scenario

Babies are normally fed milk for the first four months of life. The present recommendation is that mothers should be encouraged to breast feed their infants. Why is breast feeding best for the baby?

Some pointers

There are three proteins present in breast milk that protect the young baby from gastrointestinal and respiratory infections:

- The first is the immunoglobulin IgA. These antibodies are active against a wide range of bacterial, viral, fungal, parasitic antigens. This immunity, however, is dependent on the mother's antigenic exposure.
- The second protein is lactoferrin. This binds free iron in milk and is thought to limit this mineral to potentially pathogenic organisms in the gastrointestinal tract. The levels are high in the first week of birth and then gradually decline over the next three months.
- The third protein is lysozyme, which increases during lactation. This helps to break down bonds in the bacteria membranes and thus works synergistically with the other two proteins to protect the child.

Approximately 50 per cent of the energy in human milk is provided by fats. The fatty acid composition, however, is determined by the mother's diet. The important long-chain fatty acids for neural tissue development in the foetus and neonate are arachidonic acid and docosahexaenoic acid, and these are constantly produced in human milk. Research continues on the importance of these acids in the development of children's intelligence, behaviour and vision. There is also investigation continuing into other nutritional and hormonal factors such as taurine in the development of the retina, and in the function of conjugating bile salts (National Dairy Council 1995).

Other physiological effects of jaw and mouth development from the sucking action could be discussed.

📖 *Extend your own knowledge*

Mascarenhas *et al.* (1998) stated that growth is an extremely complex process influenced by genetics, environment, illness and nutritional status. They offered a comprehensive menu of measurements that are important in making a good nutritional assessment. They suggested that the best way to assess dietary intake is to perform a three-day weighed record of food intake, of which one day should be from school and one from the weekend. In the UK, children are eating much 'junk' food, yet they seem to be bigger and healthier and to be developing in expected ways.

Q: What comment do you have about the effect on long-term health from children's diets in their school years?

Chapter 8

The reproductive system

- Embryology of the reproductive system
- Changes in the system at birth
- Body composition and sex differences
- Body fat and sex differences
- Changes in the system at puberty
- Ovary cycle
- Menstrual cycle
- Exercise and the menstrual cycle

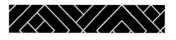

THE MOST FUNDAMENTAL and obvious difference between boys and girls lies in the anatomy and physiology of their reproductive systems. Once the exact nature and the extent of the biological sex differences are understood, the environmental influences and experiences which shape the way individual children live and the limitations that they put upon themselves can also be considered. Most small children by the age of three years will have noticed the differences between themselves and naked others, especially if they have bathed together. Many have special names for their 'different bits'. Over childhood as children grow, sex differences are evident, but the most striking changes are those occurring during puberty. Wells (1991) explains these numerous sex differences that include growth rate, skeleton, centre of gravity, pelvic bones and body composition that are brought about by development in the reproductive system.

Embryology

The final maleness/femaleness relates to the genetic sex, the gonad sex and genital sex.

In the first five weeks of gestation the foetus has an 'indifferent gonad' made up of two layers, an outer cortex and an inner medulla. If male, the medulla forms a testis (gonad sex), while the cortex disappears under the influence of the testis-determining factor on the Y chromosome (genetic sex). If no Y chromosome is present, the cortex will develop and the embryo will continue to develop as a female (Roberts and Power 1996). Sertoli cells in the testis cause Leydig cells to differentiate and produce androgens which then masculinise the embryonic genital organs (genital sex) (Dudley 1995). As the pre-Sertoli cells start to differentiate they secrete anti-Müllerian hormone which causes the Müllerian ducts (Figure 8.1), the embryonic female tract, to regress. Vines (1993) suggests, interestingly, that the effect of the Y chromosome in fact starts earlier, at conception, in order to speed up the growth of the male embryo and allow this differentiation before the oestrogen levels of the mother rise and oppose its effect. By the ninth or tenth week the Leydig endocrine cells secrete testosterone, regulated by the chorionic gonadotropin secreted by the placenta. At eight to twelve weeks testosterone will have stimulated growth of the male Wolffian system (Figure 8.1), the epididymis, vas deferens and the three accessory glands of the prostate, bulbourethral glands and the seminal vesicle, which are completed by fifteen weeks. At this time the levels of foetal testosterone are at their highest and testosterone production is stimulated more by the foetus' own pituitary gland.

The reproduction tract anatomy then develops in the male and female, although the timing of these processes differs. By the third month of gestation the female Müllerian system is developed. Fallopian tubes and their associated fimbriae, uterus and inner section of the vagina are complete.

Germ cell development also shows different time scales. In the male, the primordial cells that will produce sperm remain dormant from the seventh week of embryonic development until puberty. In the female, under the influence of two X chromosomes, the primordial germ cells undergo a few more mitotic divisions after this time to develop eggs, and begin meiotic division by the fifth month of foetal life. They then also remain dormant until puberty.

Circulating sex hormones may also affect the developing nervous system and subsequent behaviour (Carlson 1998). Androgen levels appear to have an effect on the developing brain. Eventual sexual behaviour, sexual orientation and different anatomy may all be

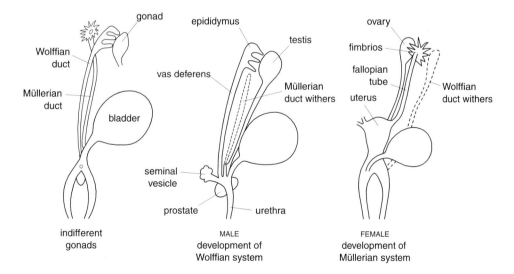

FIGURE 8.1   The Müllerian and Wolffian systems

related to the embryo's exposure to fluctuating sex hormones from its own development and that of its mother through the placenta barrier. Carlson suggests that the effects can be seen in childhood, where boys are seen to be more aggressive than girls, and in the adult, where sexual orientation may be the result of brain structure determined before birth. Research continues on the nature–nurture debate and the effect of stress hormones on the unborn child.

Changes at birth

In the male, testicles usually descend through the inguinal canal to the scrotum as the abdominal viscera grow and testosterone action increases. This descent is necessary for the later maturation of the sperm, which needs a cooler temperature, 1–2°C, than body heat. If the testicles are retained the individual may be sterile and the tubules will become fibrous, although the secondary sexual characteristics will occur as the Leydig cells which produce testosterone may still function. Some very premature male infants have undescended testicles as normally they do not descend until thirty-eight to forty weeks; these babies will have to be monitored. The undescended testes may be impalpable, abnormal, or ectopic, where they have followed the wrong route for their descent. Other anatomical aberrations result in hydroceles and hernias where there is a persistent process vaginalis, which is the pouch of peritoneum that accompanies the descent of the testes (Moules and Ramsay 1998). The seminiferous tubules are solid at birth and will not enlarge and canulize until the testicles enlarge at puberty. The adult testicle weight is forty times that of the newborn baby.

The prostate gland and the rectum are the only two major organs in the pelvis at birth. The prostate grows slowly until puberty and then doubles in size over a short period. It then continues to grow slowly for some years. The penis is relatively large in the new baby, and the prepuce imperfectly separated from the glans. The spongy tissue grows throughout childhood.

In the female, the ovaries are small at birth but large compared to testicles. They lie in the abdominal cavity in the infant and only enter the ovarian fossae at approximately six years of age as the bladder descends into the pelvis. A full complement of 400,000 eggs is present at birth in the ovary, which then declines in number over childhood. Abdominal injury, infection and drug therapy in child-hood can destroy this finite supply. The ovarian tissue will grow to twenty times its weight until puberty, when remaining egg release is stimulated by the hypothalamus. The uterus is large at birth due to the influence of maternal hormones through the placenta, and the size of the cervix is larger than the organ. It lies in the same plane as the vagina until the bladder descends at six years, when it will bend forward in the adult posture of anteversian and anteflexion (Sinclair 1991).

In both sexes the breasts may be enlarged in the period immediately after birth, and may discharge clear fluid. This is due to stimulation from the maternal hormones. This effect subsides in the first few weeks of extra-uterine life.

Body composition and sex differences

Under the influence of testosterone, males have higher body density than females at all ages and lower percentages of fat. These differences emerge at three to four years and are maintained throughout childhood. Lean body mass, which includes the essential lipid-rich stores in the bone marrow, brain, spinal cord and internal organs (Katch and McArdle 1993) increases from 25kg at ten years to 42kg at sixteen for girls, whereas muscle mass increases from about 12kg at nine years to 23kg at fifteen years. Girls attain two-thirds of this lean body mass compared to boys over this time. During puberty, under the influence of oestrogen, girls will acquire more body fat and show a different distribution.

Body fat and sex differences

In all young children the subcutaneous fat overlying the limbs is greater than over the trunk. In puberty boys lose this limb fat but gain trunk fat. In girls this change is less marked and fat accumulates specifically round the shoulders, hips and buttocks. The girls have higher amounts of essential body fat because of the tissue laid down in the breast and other sex-specific tissues. The absolute level of storage fat equals that of boys, but because the girl is lighter than the boy the relative storage fat is greater. The girl at the end of puberty will have 8–10 per cent more body fat than the boy; her sex-specific fat will be about 5 per cent of her total. However, physical activity and socio-cultural influences will produce the larger differences between both males and females (Wells 1991).

The fat of the body is contained in a specific connective tissue called adipose tissue. Fat is an energy store, but not all the stores are equally labile; subcutaneous stores are used before those round the kidney. Fat appears in the subcutaneous tissues about the sixth month of gestation and is important in temperature control of the newborn. It accounts for 25 per cent of the total weight of the baby. Pads of fat may be seen on the soles of the feet and in the cheeks of the very young. Katch and McArdle (1993) measured the fat cells of male and female pre-pubescent children in a cross-sectional study of thirty-four children. He found that the fat cell size up to one year was a quarter of the adult measurement and that it tripled in size during the first six years of life. By the age of thirteen years the cells had not changed but were still smaller than adult levels. Fat cell number trebled in the first year of life and then increased gradually up to the age of ten years. After this time there was a gradual increase of size and number to adult levels throughout puberty. Katch suggests

- that diet in pregnancy could modify this fat cell development; bottle feeding and the early introduction of solid foods could be the critical times to influence the laying down of adipose tissue.
- the encouragement of children to exercise while they are growing; thus they would lay down fewer and smaller fat cells.

Genetic factors and the underlying sex hormone effects, however, would still need to be considered in the final equation.

Brown fat

Brown fat, a quickly accessible source of energy, accumulates in the neck, round the kidneys and by the scapulae, and has a good nerve and blood supply. Its large mitochondria are regulated by thermogenin, a protein that uncouples ATP production from oxygen utilisation and thus produces heat from the substrate when the infant is exposed to cold stress. The sympathetic nervous system and various hormones also stimulate this energy expenditure. Brown fat is widely distributed round the child's body until ten years, when it is mainly found round the kidneys, suprarenals and aorta (Berne and Levy 1996; Sinclair 1991).

Changes in the reproductive system at puberty

Secondary sexual characteristics in male and female

These body changes, genital sex, occur at puberty, which is a series of events that spread over several years. Sequence and timing is individual for all the many body changes that occur, but 50 per cent of children complete the changes in three years. A critical weight has been suggested of 47kg for girls in the UK to change metabolic rate and trigger hormonal changes, but different races have different critical weights. Research by Chehab *et al.* (1997) suggests that leptin, a chemical made in adipose tissue, rises towards puberty. They suggest that that this may be a factor involved in signalling to the neuroendocrine pathways the attainment of critical fat mass, a determinant for triggering puberty. Changes usually commence with a growth spurt, which in boys can begin at ten years or as late as sixteen. The same process occurs in girls but commences approximately two years earlier.

The sex hormones, which are stimulated by the hypothalamic–pituitary–gonad axis, combine with others such as thyroxine and cortisol to activate the growth of bone and muscle (Coleman and Hendry 1995). A common hypothalamus gonad-releasing hormone (GnRH) stimulus to the pituitary gland results in the production of follicle stimulating hormone (FSH) and luteinising hormone (LH) which have different effects on the ovary and testis. In the ovary, FSH stimulates the maturation of the ovum, but in the male the production of sperm in the testes. In the ovary LH stimulates the theca cells to produce androgens that are aromatised to oestrogen, and also facilitates cholesterol to the mitochondria to be converted to progesterone. In the male, LH stimulates the Leydig cells which produce testosterone. Androgens from the adrenal cortex in both sexes stimulate the growth of axilla hair and changes in sweat and sebaceous glands, which gives so many teenagers, both boys and girls, personal problems.

The specific changes seen in boys start with growth of the testes and scrotum, followed by pubic hair. Then the growth of the penis and appearance of facial hair occur at the time of increased growth, especially of the skeleton and muscles. The voice then breaks and seminal discharge occurs as the seminal vesicles canulise.

The specific changes in girls show enlargement of the breasts, vagina and uterus, and growth of pubic hair. Menarche occurs later as growth in height and widening of the pelvic girdle occur.

Ovary cycle

The female gonad has two parts: the germ cell enclosures or follicles, and the surrounding endocrine cells that secrete steroid hormones as well as inhibin, activin, follistatin, anti-Müllerian hormone and oocyte inhibitor.

The gonad acts locally to stimulate ova development, and peripherally to

- stimulate development and function of the secondary sexual organs
- regulate secretions of the hypothalamus
- regulate sex-specific physiological function
- support the conceptus in early pregnancy

There are two types of endocrine cells in the gonads that synthesise hormones from blood cholesterol. These are the granulosa cells which surround the germ cells and produce oestrogen, and the theca cells in the ovary stroma that secrete progesterone. Both these cells when transformed to luteal cells will produce progesterone. Follicle stimulating hormone (FSH) from the anterior pituitary gland stimulates the granulosa cells to secrete oestrogen, raise the number of luteinising hormone (LH) receptors and secrete inhibin. LH, also from the pituitary gland, stimulates the theca cells to secrete androgens and cholesterol to the mitochondria and their subsequent conversion to progesterone.

Germ cells in the foetus mitose until twenty-four weeks' gestation to seven million in number. After birth from eight weeks to six months, meiosis occurs, and then these cells remain suspended in development until puberty when only 400,000 remain. Hormones from both the granulosa cells round the ovum and the theca cells in the stroma modulate ovum development and secrete directly into the blood to stimulate the secondary sexual characteristics, as gonad-releasing hormone (GnRH) levels from the maturing hypothalamus in the brain rise. They act on:

- fallopian tubes
- uterus
- vagina
- breasts
- hypothalamus
- pituitary
- adipose tissue
- liver
- kidney
- bone

The cycle hormones display three phases: the follicular, ranging from nine to twenty-three days; the ovulatory, lasting one to three days; and the luteal, lasting thirteen to fourteen days.

The follicular phase begins just after the levels of FSH and LH begin to rise from their lowest level. Twenty-four hours before the bleed FSH starts to rise and continues to rise for the first half of this phase. In the second half of the phase LH starts to rise, LH eventually reaching double the FSH levels. At the same time oestrogen levels rise gradually as the granulosa cells from the dominant follicle move into production (this eventually triggers the negative feedback system to decrease FSH production in the luteal phase).

Meanwhile, androgens increase, produced from the theca cells, which leak into the granulosa cells and are aromatised to oestrogen.

In the ovulatory phase, the LH secretion spikes, together with a smaller one of FSH. The progesterone levels rise and the ovum is expelled into the fallopian tube because the LH stimulates an inflammatory response which allows the follicle to rupture. Meiosis occurs in the ovum and the second polar body is formed. The ovum is ready for conception.

The luteal phase then occurs. Negative feedback from the corpus luteum causes FSH and LH to decline. GnRH pulses are reduced and the progesterone levels increase tenfold. Oestrogen is secreted by the corpus luteum and, if no pregnancy occurs, the oestrogen and progesterone dramatically decline and trigger GnRH release, and the bleed starts.

Menstrual cycle

Positive feedback of oestrogen levels on GnRH release in the hypothalamus is the last maturation effect, thus ovulation is not usual in the first menstrual cycles. These cycles are often irregular because the bleeding is caused by oestrogen levels falling as the Graafian follicles die before they release their ovum.

The menstrual cycle, which can be of any length from nineteen to thirty-six days, is controlled by a group of steroid hormones known collectively as the oestrogens and progesterones. It will occur two years after the commencement of secondary sexual changes, and when body mass, critical adipose mass and skeletal maturation are favourable. It is dependent on LH levels and is usual between the ages of eleven and fifteen years. Height increase stops one to two years after menses start as oestrogen closes epiphyseal plates.

The menstrual cycle is a local rhythm of the ovary and can be disrupted by situations that affect the ovary function and the function of the pituitary that stimulates and inhibits it. Calorie deprivation, habitual strenuous exercise, stress and depression have all been linked to changes in menstrual cycle function (Chrousos *et al.* 1998). Oestrogen and progesterone are released from the ovary over approximately forty years of the female fertile period: from menarche to menopause. These hormones are, in turn, controlled by hormones released from the anterior pituitary, FSH and LH. The pituitary hormones themselves are controlled by the hypothalamus hormone GnRH as FSH, LH, oestrogen and progesterone hormones, circulating in the blood throughout the monthly cycle, change. The hypothalamus, also, can be mediated by

- endorphins
- dopamine
- ACTH
- cortisone
- androgens
- thyroxine levels in the blood

Thus this hypothalamic–pituitary–gonad axis can be complex in its normal function.

Young people's cycles can be influenced by

- sleep/wakefulness
- pain
- emotion
- fright
- smell
- light
- thought

The hypothalamus position in the brain connects to all the centres of the nervous system that respond to the environment in which the individual lives.

The uterus lining shows two phases that keep it regularly prepared for conception: the proliferative phase and the secretory phase.

In the proliferative phase, the endometrium is at first thin with sparse glands which have straight, narrow lumens. The cervical mucus is scant and viscous. As oestrogen levels rise, secreted by the developing follicle in the ovary, the endometrium thickens three to five times, the glands proliferate and the spiral arteries elongate. Cervical mucus becomes copious, watery, and contains an elastic substance creating channels for sperm entry.

If no conception occurs the secretory phase commences. The progesterone levels rise, under the influence of the growing corpus luteum in the ovary, and endometrial growth stops. Glycogen in the glands moves to their lumen and is secreted in large quantities. The stroma of the uterus lining becomes oedematous and the arteries elongate and coil. The cervical mucus becomes sticky and reduces in quantity. The arteries go into spasm and release prostaglandins, which ultimately leads to tissue necrosis and cell death. This layer is then shed and menstrual flow occurs. Approximately 50ml of blood, glandular secretions and tissue fragments flow from the uterine cavity – about two tablespoons. Interestingly, the menstrual blood does not clot until it reaches the vagina because some of the clotting factors normally found in blood are destroyed by the enzymes of the uterus; the clots that appear with heavy flow are a combination of red blood cell clumps, mucus, glycogen and glycoproteins (Wells 1991).

Painful periods are a common experience in teenagers. It is this prostaglandin release that increases the inflammatory response in the myometrium to respond with muscle spasm that is so uncomfortable. There is some evidence to suggest that athletic females have less experience of painful periods and a generally better attitude towards menstruation than those who do not exercise. Some believe that regular aerobic exercise promotes menstrual health, and others that believe females who have disability from their menstrual cycle do not exercise by choice.

Figure 8.2 shows the uterine lining during the menstrual cycle.

Exercise and secondary amenorrhea

Today, some girls are exercising to professional levels and are successful in sporting careers. The effect of training on the human body is now an exact science, thus research into female body function is available. The interesting thing about the female body is that it does not respond healthily to extreme training, the most serious problem being that of bone loss when the oestrogen levels are reduced in the blood. The 'stress hormone', cortisol, is also implicated as it reduces the amount of FSH and LH to control the female ovary cycle. As muscle is built, the loss of body fat will yield less oestrogen aromatised from androgens. Thus moderate exercise is good for a girl's healthy body, but Wells (1991) and Chrousos *et al.* (1998) have demonstrated a sensitive hypothalamic–pituitary–gonad/adrenal axis to extreme conditions.

Abnormalities have been documented in female runners and

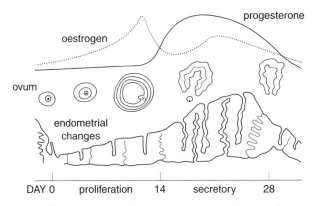

FIGURE 8.2 Uterine lining, ova changes and circulating hormones during the menstrual cycle

ballet dancers more than in swimmers and cyclists. These are characterised by low circulating oestrogens and absence of normal preovulatory increase in follicle stimulating hormone as well as a decrease in LH. This suggests that their problem lies in the hypothalamus rather than the pituitary, as artificial GnRH will stimulate a FSH response. Exercising females have also been found to experience anovulary cycles, which have a short luteal phase and abnormally low circulating progesterone and oestrogen. Dietary changes have also been implicated: amenorrheic females who do not exercise have been found to eat fewer calories and to consume less protein than their eumenorrheic sisters (Williams and Wallace 1989).

Physiology knowledge in practice

Scenario

You have been asked to talk to a group of sexually active thirteen year old girls about contraception. What would you discuss in relation to sexual activity, and what would you recommend for their contraceptive use?

Some pointers

Robert Irwin (1997), in his article on sexual health promotion and nursing, suggests that there are two characteristic dimensions of health education as practised by nurses, which are the transmission of new knowledge and the creation of a trusting relationship with clients. Further on in this article he suggests that practitioners who provide sexual health counselling must themselves be self-aware of their own value system and acceptance as a sexual being. Thus physiology knowledge must be given in a suitable environment by a confident and caring professional.

Young girls should be made aware of the development of their bodies, and that at thirteen years their internal anatomy is not yet mature. For example, the cervix at this age is still of cuboid epithelium, as the squamous epithelium has not yet covered the lower third where the penis will impinge on intercourse. The fragile entrance to the uterus is thus exposed to damage which will harbour bacterial, viral and fungal infections. If multiple partners are chosen, research has shown that they run the risk of developing cancer of the cervix later in life, as infections are carried under the prepuce of some males.

In Thompson's book, *Going All the Way: Teenager Girls' Tales of Sex, Romance and Pregnancy*, which reports on her large research project on 400 girls from different parts of the USA, she presents the impetus for intercourse as a complex urge for love, popularity, gender equality, rebellion and rights. The professional needs to be mindful of the second WHO recommendation for sexual health as 'freedom from fear, shame, guilt, false beliefs, and other psychological factors inhibiting sexual response' (1986, cited in Irwin 1997) and that these girls have a right to make choices for themselves as long as they understand the consequences of the choices they make (The Children Act 1989).

The contraceptive best suited for them is the lubricated condom. This is within their control to supply, and it offers protection from transmitted diseases. The lubrication assists the immature vagina to allow easy passage of the penis without causing irritation, soreness and trauma if vaginal secretions are not copious. It also does not interfere with their ovarian and menstrual cycles' natural rhythms that are still stabilising.

Extend your own knowledge

Woodroffe *et al.* (1993) show boys to have higher mortality rates from injury at all ages than do girls. They show, also, that the differences increase with age, the five to fourteen year old boys being twice as likely to die from accidents as girls.

Roberts and Power (1996) made a comparison of class-specific mortality in 1981–91, and found that social class five had 3.5 more deaths from accidents than social class one in children aged between one and fifteen years.

Q: What is it about the Y chromosome and the physiology of the male reproductive system that might explain Woodroffe *et al.*'s statistics and the psycho-physiology of Roberts' work?

Chapter 9

The immune system

- Protection from micro-organisms
- Acquisition of B and T cell immunity
- Embryology of the thymus
- Lymph vessel development
- Lymphocytes in the foetus and newborn
- Rhesus isoimmunisation
- Acute and chronic stress
- Chronic stress hormones
- Immunisation
- Points of interest when vaccinating children
- The future for vaccination programmes

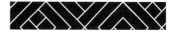

INFANTS AND SMALL children are a susceptible host group, as their immune systems require many years to develop. Before birth, the foetus is protected, to a large extent, by the placenta. Children's resistance to infection depends on their general body defence mechanisms, their innate genetic inheritance and an acquired passive or active resistance from their exposure to the world around them. Internal and external stressors can reduce their resistance to disease, and immunisation programmes through life aim to boost their ability to remain healthy and thus allow them to develop in the optimum physical condition.

Protection from micro-organisms

- Intact skin and mucosa surfaces act as the primary non-immunological host defence with the antimicrobial enzyme, lysozyme, in secretions such as sweat, tears and saliva. This enzyme helps to break down the polysaccharide cell wall of gram positive organisms. The acidity of gastric juices and the microflora in the upper respiratory tract and mouth, colon and skin also provide a protective barrier.
- Inflammation results in the vascular and cell changes that respond to the presence of dead tissue, micro-organisms, toxins and inert foreign material. The chemical mediators which trigger these events are derived from both specific cells and plasma proteins. The complement system is one of four cascades which are activated by an antigen/antibody reaction or presence of a toxin.
- Phagocytes remove unwanted material from the body. Microglia, in the brain and spinal cord, also have this function. They phagocytose the redundant cells culled in the process of brain development during the early childhood years (see Chapter 3 on the nervous system). They can later become phagocytes if nerve tissue is damaged, secreting proteases to excite the inflammatory response (Streit and Kincaid-Colton 1995).
- The immune response is activated by lymphocytes in the blood. There are two groups of lymphocytes, the B cells and the T cells. B cells produce chemicals called antibodies or immunoglobulins, whereas T cells interact directly with the invading

antigen. The immune response relies on communication with all other cellular defence systems through a complex network of receptors and mediators. However, the principal cells are the lymphocytes, which are mobile cells found in the blood, thymus, lymph nodes, spleen and tissue spaces. They require interaction with macrophages to function; these 'big eaters' secrete monokines, chemicals that alert lymphocytes, when attacking an antigen. The lymphocytes are able to differentiate between the host and antigen; produce specific antibodies for specific antigens; maintain a memory of antigen invasion; and are self-regulating to deactivate when antigens are removed from the body (see Figure 9.1).

Acquisition of immunity

Immunity is acquired in two ways. Active immunity follows exposure and stimulation of the immune response to any infection, such as the common cold and chickenpox, or by immunisation against hepatitis, measles, mumps and rubella (MMR). Passive immunity is short-lived immunity, occurring when immunoglobulins pass from the mother to the foetus across the placenta, from the mother to the baby in breast milk, or which are injected when immunocompromised children who have not been immunised are exposed to viruses such as measles (Simpson 1998).

Lymphocyte development

B cells

B cells appear in the liver a week later than T cells are identifiable. They then migrate to the bone marrow. B cells in the foetal liver differ from those found later in the bone marrow. Earlier cells make immunoglobulins (antibodies) that can bind to a wide variety of antigens but with relatively low affinity. The later cells make antibodies that react more strongly with their specific antigen nearer the time of birth. Stromal cells in the bone marrow are essential for culturing B cells; they interact with progenitor B cells by means of surface molecules. They also make soluble protein factors such as

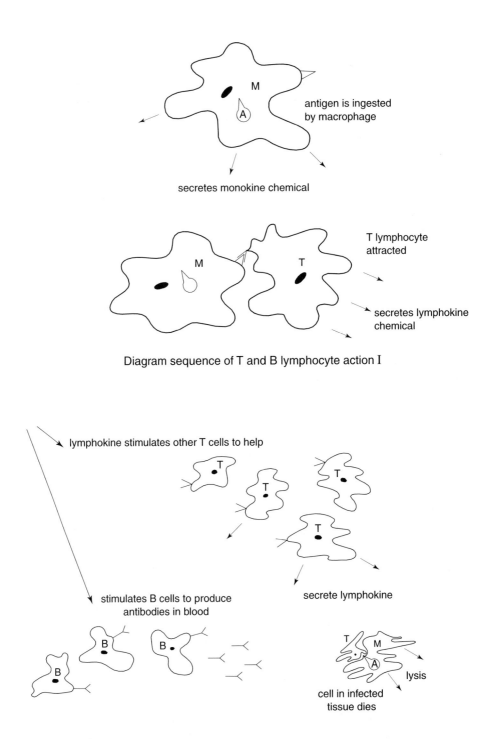

FIGURE 9.1   Sequence of T and B lymphocytes' action on antigen

interleukin seven that binds to receptors on the pro B and pre B cells, signalling them to divide and differentiate. First, they encode their genetic fragments to form immunoglobulins, then they form antigen receptors on their cell surfaces. Not all immature B cells will differentiate; they need nearby mature B cells to donate their molecular message before they can themselves mature and be released into the bloodstream (Weissman and Cooper 1993). This development appears to be genetically programmed, as they need no antigen stimulus for this activity. Over the period of a lifetime, B cells will be capable of much change in order to identify one million possible different antigens.

B cells secrete a number of immunoglobulins (antibodies):

- Five to 10 per cent are IgA, which has a half life of seven days. IgA is concentrated in the respiratory and gastrointestinal (GI) tract, for example, in saliva, tears and GI secretions. It attaches to exposed surfaces by combining with a component from the epithelial cells. Breast-fed babies appear to be protected from intestinal infection early in life.
- IgG is the major immunoglobulin found in the lymphoid follicles; it represents 75 per cent of all immunoglobulins and has the smallest structure. It recognises micro-organisms and activates complement. It passes from blood to interstitial spaces, and moves easily through the placenta to provide the foetus and newborn with maternally acquired immunity for the first three months of life. It is present in high concentrations in colostrum and breast milk. Interestingly, some cultural groups advocate the disposal of colostrum before the mother's milk 'comes in' for their newborn babies.
- IgE is the immunoglobulin involved in allergic, anaphylactic and atopic reactions. The allergic individual responds to antigen invasion by combining the allergen with IgE rather than IgG, thus it is not phagocytosed. The IgE/antigen complex, instead, then stimulates mast cells in the tissues to produce histamine. Allergens such as pollen, certain foods, drugs, dust, insect venom, moulds and animal dander can produce this effect. IgE levels are raised in sensitised children.
- IgM comprises 10 per cent of the immunoglobulins and stays in the bloodstream. It is a large molecule which reacts with foreign

antigens in the blood. It also activates complement and is the major immunoglobulin produced in infancy.

Embryology of the thymus gland and T lymphocyte development

The four pharyngeal pouches separate the branchial arches in the pharyngeal part of the foregut. It is the endoderm lining of the pouch, dorsal end, which then gives rise to the inferior parathyroid glands, whereas the ventral part gives rise to the thymus gland (Matsumura and England 1992). In the sixth gestational week, the third pharyngeal pouch pinches off from the pharynx. In weeks seven and eight, the thymic primordia, one each side, elongate and migrate caudally. As the thymus epithelium proliferates, the two thymic primordia develop from hollow tubes to solid glands. By week eight, these fuse medially. The thymus in the neonate is of a variable shape with either no lobulations, or appears bilobar or trilobar, and is located finally in the mediastinum. It is large in infancy and childhood, involuting in adult life (Groër and Shekleton 1989) (Figure 9.2).

The thymus has two functions. The first is differentiation of primitive lymphocytes into immuno-competent T cells. The second is the further expansion of antigen-stimulating T cells by the production of extracts or hormonal substances such as thymosin. T cells attack bacterial, viral, parasitic and mycotic micro-organisms,

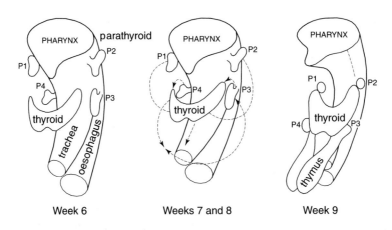

Week 6   Weeks 7 and 8   Week 9

FIGURE 9.2 Thymus development

are responsible for the auto-immune phenomena, and also participate in the rejection of malignant and transplanted cells.

T cells are thymus-derived lymphocytes which originate in the
foetal haemopoitic tissue and then migrate to the bone marrow.
They then pass to the thymus and seed in the lymph tissues of the
body over several days. By gestational week nine, lymphocytes
appear in this tissue and blood, thus the immune system is developed early in intra-uterine life. By the fifteenth week about 65 per
cent of the lymphocytes in the foetal thymus are T cells.

T cells differentiate into many different T cells in the thymus.
Here they are presented with antigens by mature cells, to which
they must react in order to survive. As they mature, they may re-
organise their genes to produce T cell receptors on their membrane
surfaces and thus become killer cells or helper/suppressor cells for B
lymphocytes.

Lymph vessel development

These vessels develop in the fifth and sixth week after conception in
a similar way to the blood vessels. Early lymph vessels join together
to form a closed network of lymphatics and lymph sacs. The six
primary lymph sacs are two jugular, two iliac, a retroperitoneal, and
one cisterna chyli which drains into the venous circulation at the
junction of the internal jugular and subclavian veins. Lymph nodes
form when mesenchymal cells migrate into the sacs and break them
up into lymph sinuses. Lymphocytes in the early lymph nodes arise
from the thymus; later some mesenchyme cells differentiate in the
nodes to also form lymphocytes. The lymph glands are present at
birth.

Lymphocytes in the foetus and newborn

B cells that synthesise immunoglobulin M (IgM) appear first,
followed by those destined to make IgG. Lymphocytes able to make
IgA appear to a limited extent near the time of birth. The presence
of these three immunoglobulins in the foetus are limited unless the
unborn baby is exposed to pathogens; then the presence of IgM may
be seen in the blood at twenty-eight weeks' gestation. However, it is

IgG that is transported across the placenta to the greatest extent, therefore this is the normal immunoglobulin profile of the newborn, even though the foetus only contributes about 5 per cent to this number. After birth these levels give protection to the baby for the first few months of life while the baby's own production rises. Premature infants may be deficient in this immunoglobulin because most of the IgG is transferred in the last trimester (Moules and Ramsay 1998). The transfer of these immunoglobulins (antibodies) depends on the structural and functional aspects of the placenta as well as the receptor-mediated mechanism, however. The rate and selectivity of transfer is also influenced by the ability of the foetal capillary endothelial cells and trophoblasts covering the chorionic villi to transport these protein structures without changing their shape. These IgG immunoglobulins reach adult levels eventually by four years of age.

Rhesus isoimmunisation occurs when the foetus red cells carry rhesus positive antigen and the mother is rhesus negative. As foetal red cells always enter the blood of the mother, the mother develops immunoglobulins against them of the IgM then IgG class. These IgG antibodies are then transported to the foetus and clump foetal red cells. This reaction is 'sensitised' by the first pregnancy, but more destructive in subsequent pregnancies as the mother responds more quickly after her body has 'learnt' to recognise this foreign structure.

Stress

It is the immune system that is most profoundly affected by the hormones released by the adrenal cortex during chronic stress. Stress is possibly a natural consequence of all children's lifestyles today, and to some extent immune deficiency will result from their exposure to chronic stressors that they perceive to be threatening. One must remember that children may see things as stressful which are not obviously so to adults: it is then the way that individual children deal with particular situations that may cause their immune system to become compromised.

Stressors can be many things for them, such as recurrent infections from repeated tonsillitis, chaotic home life or school worries.

The adrenal cortex and adrenal medulla have complementary

roles in promoting a widespread adaptation to stress: a coordinated adaptive response is mediated by the adrenal cortex's increased secretion of cortisol and the adrenal medulla's enhanced release of catecholamines (Nowak and Handford 1994).

In 'acute' stress, the cortex of the brain perceives a threatening situation and activates the autonomic nervous system sympathetic branch via the hypothalamus to release adrenaline and noradrenaline from the chromaffin cells in the adrenal medulla. These hormones circulate in the blood to prepare the body for flight. The child will look pale, sweaty and have raised alertness; metabolic rate will rise and heart rate and breathing will increase (Figure 9.3).

If the stressful situation continues, the hypothalamus activates a second system which affects the pituitary gland and its release of prolactin, growth hormone, endorphins and adrenocorticotropic hormone (ACTH), which stimulate the adrenal cortex to secrete cortisol (Figure 9.4).

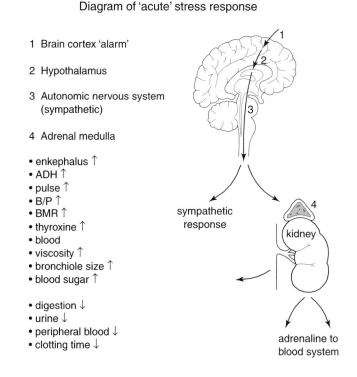

Diagram of 'acute' stress response

1 Brain cortex 'alarm'

2 Hypothalamus

3 Autonomic nervous system
  (sympathetic)

4 Adrenal medulla

• enkephalus ↑
• ADH ↑
• pulse ↑
• B/P ↑
• BMR ↑
• thyroxine ↑
• blood
• viscosity ↑
• bronchiole size ↑
• blood sugar ↑

• digestion ↓
• urine ↓
• peripheral blood ↓
• clotting time ↓

sympathetic response

kidney

adrenaline to blood system

FIGURE 9.3   The 'acute' stress response

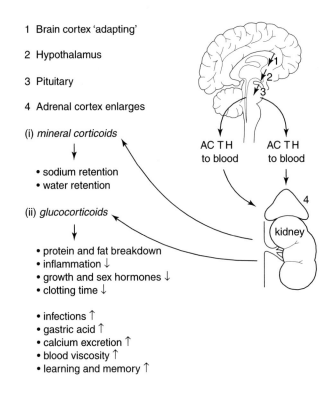

1 Brain cortex 'adapting'

2 Hypothalamus

3 Pituitary

4 Adrenal cortex enlarges

(i) *mineral corticoids*

↓

• sodium retention
• water retention

(ii) *glucocorticoids*

↓

• protein and fat breakdown
• inflammation ↓
• growth and sex hormones ↓
• clotting time ↓

• infections ↑
• gastric acid ↑
• calcium excretion ↑
• blood viscosity ↑
• learning and memory ↑

ACTH to blood   ACTH to blood

kidney

FIGURE 9.4 The 'chronic' stress response

Chronic stress hormones

- Cortisol acts as an immunosuppressant by reducing protein synthesis, including immunoglobins. It reduces peripheral blood eosinophils, lymphocytes and macrophages. Large amounts of cortisol promote atrophy of the lymphoid tissue in the thymus, spleen and lymph nodes. It directly influences the immune response to antigens. It also inhibits the production of inter-leukin one from the macrophages and interleukin two from the helper T cells. It reduces the T and B cell response and the generation of fever. However, it promotes increased energy levels as the breakdown of protein releases sugar into the blood for muscle activity and amino acids for creation of new tissue. Children who are stressed may suffer more infections than their more carefree friends, and may be underweight. Cortisol increases gastric acid secretion, which may herald the start of eating problems. It also suppresses sex hormone release: the stress of competition for the child gymnast combined with the training and muscle building all result in delayed reproduction development in the young female.

- Endorphins, secreted with ACTH, come from the pituitary and central nervous system. They regulate the production of ACTH, produce a reduced sensitivity to pain and a raised feeling of excitement. One could ask whether it is this chemical that allows children to become 'numb' and distance themselves from frightening circumstances, those children who are 'too quiet' or 'too wild'. Is this how abused children cope?

- Growth hormone, produced by the pituitary gland, will rise after the stress of physical exercise, and also with psychological stimulus. Children who are active, interested and sleep well will grow. Growth hormone is also stimulated by watching violent films (McCance and Heuther 1998). However, for each individual child there will be a point when the excitement turns into distress and reduces the production of this hormone. When this happens, lymphocyte function is disrupted and the immune response less effective.

- Prolactin acts as a second messenger for interleukin two, and normally increases B cell activation and differentiation. It is reduced in prolonged stress, especially from physical injury. Children are thus vulnerable to this stressor as they frequently have accidents at all ages.

Children's responses to stress begin prenatally and develop more fully as the child interacts with the environment. Their response to any stressor is individual: some children are more adaptive than others. Frydenberg (1997) suggests that the child's individual disposition, family warmth and having positive models to identify with are important in learning coping strategies. The child requires the carer to respond to unique cues: demanding behaviour, failure to attain 'milestones' and failure to thrive are signs of stress in the very young. The preschool child may become incontinent, have night terrors and become aggressive. The school-aged child may refuse to go to school and fall behind in studies, and the adolescent may worry about his or her changing body, heightened sexuality, peer pressure and parental discord. Challenges that are appropriate will stimulate the child to move on to the next stage of their physical competence, whereas inappropriate stressors will result in a slower rate or more dysfunctional development (Arnold 1985).

Immunisation

In the 1980s the then Health Education Council of England and Wales stated that having children immunised against whooping cough would help wipe out the disease in the population, and noted that playing on society's social conscience would increase the uptake of this vaccination (Dyson 1995). Vaccination programmes have traditionally been a national responsibility. However, with the advent of new vaccines for seventy-five infectious diseases (Katz 1997) parents, perhaps, need to be properly informed rather than morally cajoled before they present their offspring for more and more recommended injections. In the USA, children cannot access education without their vaccinations being up to date, yet in the UK where vaccination is free, not all children are protected (Riley *et al.* 1991).

The WHO European Region's 'Health For All' campaign states that by the year 2000 there should be no indigenous polio, neonatal tetanus, diphtheria, measles, or congenital rubella syndrome. In 1999 in the UK, we are not quite on target; the principal reasons, suggested by Riley *et al.* (1991) being that in inner cities families move around frequently, some mothers 'never get round to it', and some young children have frequent infections and are not considered well enough to be vaccinated. There is protection available for nine infectious diseases in the UK: diphtheria, measles, polio, tetanus, pertussis, rubella, mumps and haemophilus influenza type B infections (Hib), and tuberculosis (BCG) (DOH 1996). In 1994 uptake of these vaccines was at an all-time high, but with only the sporadic occurrence of these infections in 1998, many carers have become more concerned with the side-effects of the injections rather than morbidity of contracting the disease, so consequently uptake is falling (Moules and Ramsay 1998).

Vaccination stimulates the immune system in a variety of ways without the need of the individual to suffer the condition:

- Live but weakened (attenuated) pathogenic micro-organisms stimulate the body to recognise a foreign (antigen) protein and produce antibodies to destroy it. The memory created protects the child from future invasion of the particular pathogen. MMR vaccine can induce a mild form of measles within ten days of vaccination and/or a general inflammatory response.
- Dead organisms can be injected which have the 'shape' of the antigen but cannot divide and multiply in the body. The lymphocytes recognise them as foreign and respond, again producing a memory cell of the 'shape' for future attacks. Typhoid and pertussis (whooping cough) are commonly used in vaccination programmes. A new acellular vaccine for pertussis is available which, it is hoped, will produce a less severe reaction yet give protection from future infection.
- Toxoids, such as those from tetanus and diphtheria, are the modified bacterial toxin that has been made non-toxic, but which retains the ability to stimulate the formation of antibodies (Wong 1999).

Table 9.1 details the recommended UK immunisation schedule.

TABLE 9.1 Recommended immunisation schedule for the UK

2 months	polio, HIB, diphtheria, tetanus, whooping cough
3 months	polio, HIB, diphtheria, tetanus, whooping cough
4 months	polio, HIB, diphtheria, tetanus, whooping cough
12–15 months	measles, mumps, rubella (MMR)
3–5 years	measles, mumps, rubella (MMR), diphtheria, tetanus, polio
10–13 years	tuberculosis (BCG) (sometimes given shortly after birth)
14–19 years	diphtheria, tetanus, polio

Source: Moules and Ramsay 1998

Points of interest when vaccinating children

- If a viral vaccine is to be used, it will not be effective if the child has a viral infection such as the common cold. Inferon will be present in the bloodstream, which will inhibit the body's response to the vaccine.
- If oral polio vaccine is given to a child with a gastrointestinal infection such as diarrhoea and vomiting, the vaccine will be passed out of the gut and not completely absorbed. Even after successful polio vaccination, children will 'shed' the virus in their faeces for six weeks.
- Some viruses are cultured for vaccines in egg tissue with anti-biotics that suppress bacterial contamination. Some children may be hypersensitive and produce an allergic response to these foreign proteins, and release histamine into the tissues (Campbell 1992).
- The measles vaccine is given after one year, as the residual maternal IgG will destroy the organism before it has elicited a response. Aaby *et al.* (1995) found that the measles vaccine acti-vates the immune system in a non-specific way which provides protection against other diseases. However, recently there has been much publicity speculating that this particular vaccine is responsible for children developing Crohn's disease and autism, which is not currently supported by research (Rejtman 1998).

The future

A move to mucosal immunisation will be more economical and provide less risk of needle contamination. The use of plant engi-neering may provide fruit, such as the banana, as the vehicle for vaccine. These advances will be reliant on political will and available resources. Vaccination of pregnant women in the third trimester, when IgG can be transported across the placenta to the unborn infant, could protect against tetanus. Vaccines for sexually trans-mitted diseases would protect young teenagers who have high-risk behaviour (Katz 1997).

Physiology knowledge in practice

Scenario

A group of mothers are debating whether to have the MMR injection for their fifteen month old children. Some suggest they want their children to suffer the diseases if they catch them, as they feel the immunity will thus be better – more natural. Others want the vaccine separated into three so that their children receive immunisation for one disease at a time. How would you support their views physiologically?

At present in the UK, the MMR is taken up by the majority of families, so the 'herd' is protected and measles, mumps and rubella are infrequently seen. Thus the unvaccinated children will have a good chance of not contracting these infections, and if they do, they have a good chance that they will contract them after infancy when they have a more developed immune system and stronger physical resources to deal with them. Social and health resources are good today and the environment is hygienic. There is informed medical support for sick children everywhere in the country.

When the body is invaded by a foreign protein, i.e. an attenuated infective antigen such as measles, the immune response is first of a general nature where the body temperature rises in the inflammatory phase. Lymphocytes then develop antibodies and eventually the invading antigen is overcome and the child recovers. If the body is invaded by three foreign proteins, the immune response will have to develop three different antibody types, thus the system may have to work three times as hard and exhaust the natural resources of the child at fifteen months. Some mothers may consider rubella to be such a minor illness that they do not want a vaccination; they may be ignorant of the devastating effects this virus has on the foetus in the first trimester of pregnancy.

Extend your own knowledge

In the *Daily Telegraph* of 30 December 1998, the editorial comment on page 21 analysed government plans to reduce schoolgirl pregnancies. Britain is known to have the highest teenage pregnancy rate in Europe: 87 per cent of 41,700 babies born to fifteen to nineteen year olds were outside marriage, compared to 10 per cent in Japan. Petosa (1989, in Shucksmith and Hendry 1998) suggests the 'problem' should be addressed through ensuring supportive and yet challenging environments for these young girls, rather than prescribing more and more restrictions for them.

Q: How could you justify Petosa's stance from a physiological angle as a stress-reducing strategy?

Chapter 10

Coordinating the systems

- Thyroid gland effect in growth
- Screening
- Foetal growth
- The school-age child milestones
- Vision
- Hearing
- Weight
- Height
- The role of the thyroid
- Thyroid hormones
- The importance of the hypothalamus
- The happiness factor
- Children's emotions

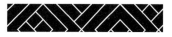

T HE MEASUREMENT OF height, weight, sight and hearing are impor- tant in child health screening because normal development ensures that children will have the best opportunity to maximise their genetic potential for life. Problems can often be addressed at an early age; if these problems are left undetected they may lead to unnecessary restriction of innate ability.

Thyroid gland effect in growth

One gland of the endocrine system is particularly important in promoting this growth in childhood: the thyroid gland, which is situated at the front of the neck, beneath the larynx. Thyroid hormones affect the use of energy and production of heat, and stimu- late linear growth, development and maturation of bone. They have critical effects, particularly on the development of the nervous system and the regulation of the reproductive system in both males and females. The thyroid is part of a network of glands controlled by the hypothalamus or 'master gland', a small area of brain tissue deep inside the skull. It is this close coordination that occurs in the hypothalamus between the nervous and endocrine systems that ensures children develop normally and maintain their finely tuned homeostasis. The interaction of the body with the brain and of the brain with the body systems must always be at the front of our minds when assessing children, as behaviour is often the only 'symptom' of an unhappy child who is not thriving.

Screening

Effective screening in child health is being updated regularly, and calls are being made for a coordinating body to oversee public health for children. There appears to be a need for professionals from health and education to work together so that effective use is made of advancing technology, and support is given to the indirect intervention by parents and teachers (Hall 1996; Robinson 1998).

Foetal growth

Measurement of foetal growth and expected dates for delivery occupy the minds of clinicians who wish to reduce the number of induced labours that increase risk to the foetus. Backe and Nakling (1998) suggest, however, that if intervention is not necessary, pregnant women can do perfectly well without accurate dating of term predictions or sizing from ultrasound. The 'average' time for a pregnancy appears to be 283 days from the last menstrual period, although it is suggested to be better practice that women are given a time interval for the expected date of labour rather than a fixed point, because predicting the length of individual pregnancies is not yet an exact science. Steer (1998) points out that it is in the mother's interests to restrict foetal growth in late pregnancy in order to increase the success of a vaginal delivery. Interestingly, this is in direct opposition to the interest of the foetus, which will want to maximise birth weight to ensure its viability. Wheeler *et al.* (1998), in a study of foetal fingerprint patterns and disproportionate intra-uterine growth, found that the high ratio of head to abdominal circumference, suggesting intra-uterine growth retardation, correlated to high numbers of whorls on the babies' fingertips. They suggest that in week ten and twelve of gestation, if cranial redistribution of blood is compromised, swelling of the fingertips may occur and a corresponding increase in whorls develop. They also suggest that the anatomical origins of the right and left subclavian arteries lead to the increase of whorls on the right hand in these same infants. Could this fingerprinting be a novel assessment of foetal growth in the future?

Rudolf and Levene (1999) set out a child surveillance programme from newborn to fourteen years. The infant and preschool child requirements, as they suggest, are as follows:

- Newborn – screening for hips, testicular descent, red reflex, phenylketonuria (after seventy-two hours' feeding), thyroid, hearing (if high risk). General examination for weight, length, head circumference and full physical examination. Health education for feeding, baby care, crying and sleep problems, and car seats.
- Ten days – screening for hips, general examination for weight

and prolonged jaundice, and health education support for nutrition, immunisation, safety and passive smoking.

- Six to eight weeks – screening of hips, general examination of weight, head circumference, eyes and development. Health education topics included are nutrition, immunisation, recognition of illness in babies and accident prevention in the home.
- Six to nine months – screening of hips, testicular descent, distraction test for hearing, and eyes for squints. Health education, again on accident prevention for choking, burns, falls, safety gates and car seats; nutrition, teeth, passive smoking and developmental needs.
- Eighteen to twenty-four months – screening of hips, haemoglobin and general examination of gait and language. Accident prevention would now cover topics such as falls from heights, drowning, poisoning and road safety. Nutrition is again discussed, as are developmental needs, language use, play and behaviour.
- Thirty-six to forty-eight months – screening of cardiac function and general examination of height and weight is suggested. A check is made on medical or developmental problems that might interfere with future education plans.

The school-aged child

Webb (1998) sets out some core activities for a school nurse:

The five year old

- structured school entrant health interview with parent
- visual acuity (Snellen chart)
- hearing (sweep test)
- discussion with teacher on any concerns

The seven to eight year old

- visual acuity
- height and weight

- general health check and check on diet and dental care

The eleven to twelve year old

- visual acuity
- height and weight
- general health check to include teenage counselling

The fourteen year old

- general health check to include self-referral for help
- questionnaire to pupil and parent for communication on health surveillance

Schools are only required to facilitate routine schoolchild health surveillance and immunisation programmes. Lightfoot and Bines (1997) suggest this gives school nurses difficulty in focusing their resources on need, and giving children access to their services. Bagnell (1995) identified many areas for negotiated screening that would change a task-orientated role to a dynamic service addressing the 'Health of the Nation' targets, such as: encouraging exercise for cardiovascular health; addressing behaviours that lead to cancer such as smoking and drinking to excess; supporting coping mechanisms for anxiety and depression; advising on sexual health and the avoidance of unwanted pregnancy; and educating children on risk-taking, with particular focus on road safety.

Vision

Preschool vision screening has been offered in most health districts in the UK for the past twenty years. Today, conflicting interpretations of reports from the USA and the UK are casting doubt as to its merit. Amblyopia, strabismus (squint) and refractive errors are the ophthalmic errors commonly seen in only 6 per cent of children and are relatively easy to treat. Rahi and Dezateux (1997) suggest that the benefits of interventions when children are seen to have problems are often under-researched and do not support the service provided, at present, for the total child population. All children are vision screened at five years when they enter full-time education, so an earlier test needs to be justified. Amblyopia is the reduced visual acuity in one eye causing different images to be received by the retina and visual cortex and eventual loss of response by the brain to the stimulus. Squint usually results from muscle imbalance of the extra-ocular muscles, which then results in the light being focused away from the fovea of the retina, thus not stimulating the reception of colour and accurate images. Refractive errors can be the outcome of eyeball size, often genetically inherited. Children are normally short-sighted at birth, but poor sight at school will hinder development both in the classroom and in outdoor pursuits.

Hearing

The earliest screening occurs by the parent, who will report the hearing baby as being startled by loud noise and calmed by and responding to a familiar voice. Milestones include the six month old baby as being able to turn the head to quiet distraction and 'babble' a range of sounds. By one year the first words should be heard and from then the development of language will occur (Bysshe 1994). However, with the availability of new technology, earlier screening is now possible to ensure children with hearing deficits are treated, because early intervention has been shown to make a significant difference to their eventual language ability and successful education.

New proposals for a neonatal hospital-based universal hearing test for all babies within a few days of birth are being made. Up to now, health visitors have carried out a distraction test in the community. However, it has been shown that the sensitivity of this distraction test varies between 18 and 88 per cent, and the electronic probe provides a better 80–100 per cent result at half the cost in manpower (Sadler 1998). The transient evoked otoacoustic emission (TEOAE) records cochlear hair cell activity in the normally functioning ear. The screening for normal hearing has usefully been incorporated by health visitors into an assessment of the parent–child relationship, but the environment in which they perform their distraction test may often have been inappropriate. It is suggested that with distracting noises and lights, tests carried out by personnel with poorly updated skills may not be reliable. Watkin and Jeremiah

(1998), however, in their evaluation of the use of the newer screening tool in Camden and Islington from 1992, support the continuing surveillance role of health visitors at the new birth visit or six-week examination, and their involvement in discussing hearing testing with parents. They also support the importance of the health visitor's assessment if later language development is poor or the child suffers recurrent ear infections.

Weight

The body mass index (weight in kg/height in metres squared) is used to determine an adult person's fatness. Some individuals, who are very muscular, can be wrongly identified; but the measurement is helpful in health screening. Underweight will be below 18.5, ideal 18.5–24.9, overweight 25.0–29.9, obese (1) 30.0–34.9, obese (2) 35.0–39.9, obese (3) 40+.

Unfortunately, these measurements are not appropriate for young children in whom the fiftieth percentile shows profound changes from birth to adult status. The child from six to twelve years doubles in weight from about 21kg to 40kg, but the body proportions change as the skeleton lengthens and fat is redistributed. The Child Growth Foundation (1994) publishes charts which include nine centile curves based on divisions of two-thirds of a standard deviation, which can be used for all children in the UK. The charts are separate for boys and girls, although the differences are very small. Must *et al.* (1991) give examples of these centile charts for children in the USA (see Table 10.1), but worldwide standardisation is more difficult as different races show different patterns of body mass changes at different ages. Secular trends will also cause difficulties over time; as populations become more affluent their children may grow heavier. A third problem is to decide when a child is too fat or too thin, for growth spurts occur at many stages from birth to adult size (Prentice 1998). Interesting work by Niinikoski *et al.* (1997) investigating growth and energy intake in children under three years showed that that lean children (5th percentile) had the highest energy intake compared to children with weight in the 50th and 95th percentile. They concluded that parental height and body mass index predicted the best growth patterns for this age range rather than weight alone.

157

Height

After the second year of life, growth hormone becomes the controller of growth rate rather than nutrition. In the adolescent, a combined effect with sex steroids speeds growth through puberty. The end point height is the most important for children; thus today, growth hormone treatment is available early for all children who show changes towards too high or too small stature which is different to their genetically predicted size (Brook 1997). The 'end point' in 1995 was 1.5cm taller than in the 1970s when the Tanner and Whithouse charts were constructed for use nationally. The new charts published by the Child Growth Foundation (Hulse 1995) are designed from cross-sectional data of 25,000 children collected from 1978–90 and take into consideration all the regional differences from the United Kingdom at that time. They have nine instead of seven centile ranges and are recommended for use at eighteen months, three years, five years, and four more measurements before the age of nine years. Ethnic minorities, again, need to be considered with caution: black children tend to be taller and have longer legs than white children. Referral is required for those individuals who cross one major centile band between five to nine years and for two major bands before this age. Those children who show height/weight discrepancy over three centile bands should also be assessed for growth and dietary history.

TABLE 10.1 Body mass index (BMI) expressed as percentile

	Centiles				
	5th	*15th*	*50th*	*85th*	*95th*
Males 11 years	15	16	17	20	24
Males 14 years	16	17	19	23	27
Males 17 years	17	19	21	25	29
Females 11 years	15	16	18	21	25
Females 14 years	16	17	19	24	28
Females 17 years	17	18	20	25	30

Source: Must *et al.* 1991

The role of the thyroid in all tissue development

The thyroid gland develops from an invagination of the tongue endoderm and migrates to a ventrocaudal location. It appears late in the fourth week as a small solid mass, and in the fifth week consists of lateral lobes connected by an isthmus (Figure 10.1). It descends to its final position, inferior to the cricoid cartilage of the larynx by the seventh week. It begins to incorporate iodine into thyroid hormones (thyroxines) and to secrete these into the blood circulation at about week ten to twelve of gestation.

The ultimobranchial body then arises from the fourth pharyngeal pouch and fuses with the thyroid gland to give rise to the parafollicular cells (C cells) that secrete calcitonin and somatostatin.

Thyroid hormones

- Calcitonin lowers serum calcium levels by inhibiting bone reabsorption and promoting bone formation by the osteoblasts. Berne and Levy (1996) suggest that this hormone is important in bone development in the foetus, but suggest that parathyroid

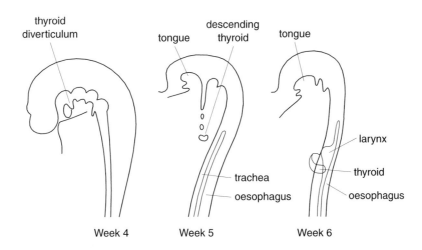

FIGURE 10.1 Migration of thyroid gland in weeks 4, 5 and 6

hormone and vitamin D are more important in the development of children's bones after birth.

- Thyroxine (T3 and T4) is regulated through a negative feedback loop involving the hypothalamus, anterior pituitary and thyroid gland. T3 and T4 show a diurnal variation, with a peak availability during late evening. These hormones require iodine for their formation: this mineral naturally occurs in fish, it may be added to other foods such as salt and is present in various amounts in the soil in which food crops grow. Thyroid hormones are degraded in the liver, kidney and skeletal muscle.

Table 10.2 shows normal serum levels of triiodothyronine in childhood.

Thyrotropin-releasing hormone (TRH) is synthesised and stored in the hypothalamus before being released into the hypothalmus-pituitary portal system and thus to the anterior pituitary. Here, thyrotropin (thyroid stimulating hormone, TSH) is released to the blood circulation where it is taken up by the thyroid gland. The process of iodine trapping and of thyroxine (T3 and T4) synthesis is stimulated or repressed by the presence or absence of this hormone. It also increases glucose oxidation and nucleic acid, protein, and phospholipid synthesis. These actions underlie this hormone's growth-promoting effects on the thyroid gland. Its secretion is controlled in the anterior pituitary by changes in thyroxine levels of only 10–30 per cent in the blood. It is inhibited by dopamine and somatostatin produced in the hypothalamus, and by cortisol and growth hormone.

In fasting, the hypothalamus and pituitary function are reduced,

TABLE 10.2 Normal serum levels of triiodothyronine, total T3-RIA in childhood

Cord	0.46–1.08 nmol/l
	1.16–4.00 nmol/l
1–5 years	1.54–4.00 nmol/l
5–10 years	1.39–3.70 nmol/l
10–15 years	1.23–3.23 nmol/l
Adult	1.77–2.93 nmol/l

Source: Wong 1996

thyroxine levels fall and resting metabolic rate is decreased. Energy is conserved for vital body activities, growth will slow and brain function will become sluggish. Children who have too few calories are lethargic and lack concentration and interest in their surroundings. Thyroxine is an insulin antagonist; it stimulates the secretion of glycogen to release glucose into the bloodstream, it enhances hormone effect to increase appetite and increase absorption of glucose from the gastrointestinal tract, lipid breakdown, and generally accelerates the metabolic response to starvation (Berne and Levy 1996).

In exposure to cold, pituitary TSH increases to stimulate thyroxine production and the use of energy. Neonates show a raised plasma TSH and thyroxine level for several weeks as they move from the maternal to external environment (Berne and Levy 1996). Perhaps this is another of the reasons why the new baby shows a weight loss, together with a 'drying out' and adjustment to feeding schedules. Children appear to be more hungry in the cold winter months and enjoy a carbohydrate-rich diet. In a cold environment, such as playing in the snow for a morning, they may become tired more quickly than when they play outside in the summer months.

Thyroxine enters all body cells by carrier-mediated transport and influences the nucleus to increase synthesis of proteins. It is especially important for growth of the central nervous system and cerebration in the first two years of life. It increases respiratory rate and oxygen consumption, red cell mass and calorie use:metabolic rate (BMR). Body temperature then rises and alterations occur in blood flow to the skin, sweating and ventilation to control this change. Cardiac output, force and rate is increased as this hormone increases myocardial calcium uptake and enzyme activity. Muscle tone and vigour also improve. Systolic blood pressure rises as output increases, and diastolic blood pressure reduces as peripheral vessels dilate due to increased tissue metabolism.

Food is broken down more quickly and wastes are more rapidly excreted under its influence. Tissues become more sensitive to sympathetic nervous system stimulus. Neurones, which also terminate on the blood vessels in the thyroid gland, produce neurotransmitters which may directly affect its secretory activity stimulated by the hypothalamus and cerebrum. Anxiety and stress may result in this mechanism being activated. Thyroxine stimulates skeletal height and development, and maturation of the bone and teeth. It acts directly on the chondrocytes in the growth plate and stimulates the secretion of growth hormone (see Chapter 2 on the skeletal system).

The importance of the hypothalamus in linking the physical with the psychological person

The hypothalamus develops (Figure 10.2) from the same structure as the cerebral hemispheres and olfactory tracts. The thalamus and hypothalamus differentiate by the end of the sixth gestational week. The thalamus acts primarily as a relay centre for the cerebral cortex from all areas of the body; the hypothalamus regulates the endocrine activity of the pituitary as well as many reflex autonomic nervous responses. The hypothalamus also participates in the limbic system which controls emotion and sexual behaviour, the sleep/wake states, food and water intake and regulation of the immune system.

The endocrine function of the hypothalamus is as a central relay station for collecting and integrating signals from the thalamus, reticular activating substance, the limbic system, the eyes and the cortex. It will then influence the pituitary function to change sleep/wake cycles, pain, emotion, fright, smell, light and thought (Berne and Levy 1996).

It will directly affect the coordinating of sexual behaviour. In

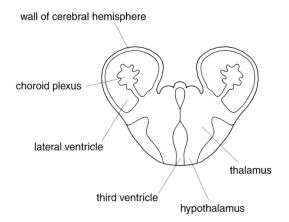

Figure 10.2 Hypothalamus development at foetal week ten

stressed females, the hypothalamic function of corticotropin-releasing hormone (CRH) activates the adreno-cortico-trophic hormone (ACTH) and inhibits gonadotropin-releasing hormone, growth hormone and sexual activity. The glucocorticoids released in the stress response suppress leutinising hormone and thus ovulation, reduce the production of ovarian oestrogen and progesterone, and render target cells resistant to oestradiol (Chrousos *et al.* 1998). Teenage girls may, then, present with amenorrhagia if they are anxious about exams, worried about their social life or unsure of their relationship with parents and family. Pregnancy, however, may need to be discounted first.

Through its interhypothalamic axonal connections, the hypothalamus produces a pituitary response to changes in the autonomic nervous response, temperature regulation, water balance (see renal system) and energy requirements. For example, thyroid hormones T3 and T4 will increase metabolic rate, the use of glucose by the cells and heating of the body. The neurons that regulate thyroid hormone release in the hypothalamus lie conveniently close to those that regulate appetite and temperature control (see Chapter 3 on the nervous system and Chapter 7 on the digestive system). Table 10.3 shows the interrelationship of hypothalamic functions.

The happiness factor

The state of being 'happy' is perhaps difficult to define, but more obvious when it is experienced or observed. Having a happy emotion may be a very different 'thing' for every child; that adults think they are able to share their happiness may be an illusion. To experience an emotion one needs first to be able to perceive the world outside and be in a context to feel.

Perception requires the sense organs which are regulated by a nervous system and a memory check to relate experiences against one another. It would be interesting to compare the perceptions of children with learning disability with those who are blind and those who are deaf. It is interesting, also, to ask whether one can perceive one's world at different levels; for example, the children who are drugged – with Ritalin for attention deficit hyperactivity disorder (ADHD) or with Piriton for hay fever control. Babies may be more perceptive than is thought, as they experience relatively more light

TABLE 10.3 Chart showing the interrelationship of hypothalamic functions

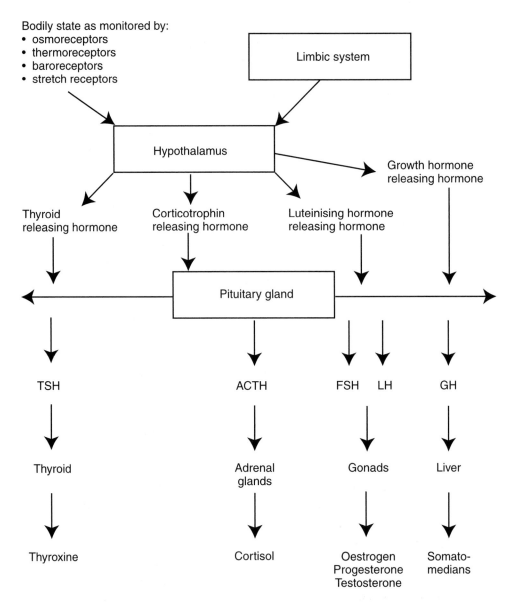

Source: Adapted from Berne and Levy 1996

sleep than older children. Adolescents may be perceiving many things at once on different levels when they do their homework, listen to music, have the cat on their lap and chew gum.

The context in which children learn to perceive is of equal

importance to their ability to perceive. It is generally considered that a caring home is vital for stable emotional development. If this is so, a context such as that experienced by abused children or war victims will jeopardise the child's chance to be happy but this is not always found to be so. Mussen (1990) shows that the biggest causes of sadness for four to seven year old children are interpersonal and environmental events: thus the context of their perceptions is important.

If awareness is at different levels, then emotions may also be at different levels; the cortical effect may be altered to respond to the child's changing ability to understand and cope. The hypothalamus, as it matures, may subtly balance messages from the cortex through to the endocrine and nervous system, thus keeping emotional response under some control. One could interpret Freud's 'id', 'ego' and 'superego' in this way and see the two year old's temper tantrum as a learning of this system. It is interesting to speculate whether the foetus feels emotion towards its mother's womb, and whether this is happiness. Gross (1996) cites Cannon, the physiologist who first described homeostasis, who suggests that one cannot have specific physiology for every emotion and that physiological change may not always cause an emotion. Cannon suggests that emotion can occur without physiological change and that it can be sudden, whereas many visceral responses may be slow. However, Mussen describes both the psychology and physiology as vital to the equation of having an emotion. He describes four components of the phenomenon:

- *The context that produces the emotion.* Children can be affected by different situations to adults; happiness for a child may be when they are absorbed in acquiring some new skill.
- *The physiological change.* Experiences of sympathetic activity and adrenaline flow such as 'a warm glow', 'shiver through my spine' and 'sick with fear' are expressed in stimulating situations. Children may sleep well and have increased appetite as their parasympathetic system is activated and they feel content, drowsy and safe.
- *The emotional communication*, be it visual, verbal or body movement. This is perhaps the easiest one to measure in most children, because many smile readily. It can, however, be

misconstrued in the child who always smiles but gradually stops demanding attention. This child may actually be sad.

- *The emotional experience.* If the child has enjoyed being happy and has experienced it enough to recognise it, the child will know what it is to be happy. Perhaps, at the end of the day, if the experience is 'good' for children one can say they are happy.

Papalia and Olds (1992) suggest that emotion is a fundamental element of personality, therefore the ability to be happy may be genetically determined. Babies, at birth, show different awareness, feed more or less hungrily, respond to handling differently, tolerate their wet nappy for various lengths of time, sleep in particular positions and respond to noise with more or less equanimity.

Context, however, will then be a powerful part of the equation: a child who is surrounded by happiness has a good chance to develop the ability to be happy to a larger or lesser extent.

Physiology knowledge in practice

Scenario

A group of mothers are discussing the heights of their two year old daughters. There seems to be an expectation that the girls should be smaller than the boys. The mothers of the girls are worried that the children will eventually reach a height of over six feet tall, a height they consider to be a disadvantage for a female in the UK. They have calculated this projected height with reference to Bee (1995), who directs the reader to double the child's height at two years to find an estimate of their adult measurement. What would explain this estimation of height in children?

Some pointers

- The first question is to ask if these children were measured *on* their second birthday. At this age children are growing at approximately 7–11cm per year, so if, at the time of measurement, one was two years and two days and another two years and eight months, the elder child may have had much more time to grow.

- Growth in childhood is not a steady increase; children seem to grow fatter before they grow taller – the 'Christmas tree' phenomenon. The girls may have been measured at a 'fat' stage or a 'spurt' stage.
- Height as a percentage of predicted adult height at the age of two years is 52 per cent for girls and 50 per cent for boys. Thus the girls in a group of two year old children may very well be taller.
- The predicted height is normally genetically governed, allowing for the secular trends which have effect over generations. The height of both the *biological* parents should be averaged and the mid-parental height calculated (MPH). Seven centimetres should then be taken from this MPH for a girl's predicted adult height. The target centile range (TCR) will lie between the 91st and 9th measurements + 8.5cm, assuming the parents are within 'normal' height ranges themselves.

Extend your own knowledge

Q: From Webb's (1998) suggestions on schoolchild screening, what would you include in the questionnaire for the older children, and how would you follow it up using your physiology knowledge?

Glossary

atheroma Deposition of lipids and other substances in the intima (inner layer) of the medium and large arteries. This then becomes thickened. Smooth muscle cells, collagen and elastic fibres accumulate and lipids, especially cholesterol, deposit on the artery wall, narrowing its lumen.

bifurcation To fork or lead into two pathways.

chondroitin sulphate The organic matrix of bone imparts its tensile strength. Ninety-five per cent of this matrix is collagen with hyaluronicacid and chondroitin sulphate constituting 5 per cent. The mineral matrix consists of amorphous calcium phosphate and a crystalline structure like hydroxyapatite.

cytoplasm Cellular substance between the plasma membrane and the nuclear membrane. It typically contains proteins, organic polyphosphates, nucleic acids and other ionised substances that cannot permeate the plasma membrane. The majority of these impermeant intracellular ions are negatively charged at physiological pH.

dendrites Neuron cytoplasm processes which increase the surface area of the nerve cell body to be available for connections to other nerve bodies.

desquamated epithelium The shed lining (epithelium) of the gut.

genioglossus muscle A triangular muscle attached by a short tendon to the inner surface of the mandible symphysis. It spreads out in a fan-like form to attach to the hyoid bone, muscles of the pharynx and the whole length of the under surface of the tongue. This muscle draws the tongue forward and protrudes the apex through the mouth. It draws the middle of the tongue down to make the upper surface concave from side to side.

glomerular filtration The process where fluid from the blood is forced under pressure out of tiny capillaries (the glomerulus) in the kidney into tiny tubes (the nephron) where reabsorption of substances useful to the body such as sugar are reabsorbed and waste products such as urea are carried out of the kidney to the ureter and bladder for excretion.

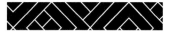

human genome   The human genome is the chemical structure of all 46 chromosomes in a human cell nucleus.

hyperpyrexia   (or fever) This is when the body temperature rises to a level where cell metabolism is disrupted. Many centres would consider 39° as a measurement at which to initiate antipyretic medication.

hypothalamus   or 'master gland'. A small area of brain tissue deep inside the skull.

intermediate mesoderm   A layer of cells between the endoderm and ectoderm which differentiates in the first stage of embryo development. It develops into the connective tissues, teeth, muscles, circulatory and lymph systems, urogenital tract and the endothelial linings of the pericardial, pleural and peritoneal cavities.

kernicterus   This is caused by damage to cells in the basal ganglia of the brain due to excessive accumulation of bilirubin in the blood plasma after birth. The child develops motor difficulties in all parts of the body. It is seen when the child tries to initiate movement under voluntary control. Limbs jerk, facial expression distorts and speech is irregular.

lipoprotein   Transport of non-polar lipids (fats) in plasma requires that they are joined with a protein. This occurs in the liver. The protein part of the lipoprotein then serves catalytic functions and interacts with specific cell receptors to facilitate endocytosis of fat into the cells.

metabolic alkalosis   This is when the body fluids' pH rises above neutral (pH 7.45) and becomes alkaline. The bicarbonate ions in the blood increase. It is different to respiratory alkalosis where blood carbon dioxide (which is relative to its acidity) is reduced. This occurs in conditions of overbreathing where carbon dioxide from the lungs is lost in excess of inhalation of oxygen.

mitochondria   Small organelles in the cell cytoplasm. They are the site of aerobic cellular respiration. ATP (adenosine triphosphate) is produced in them which stores energy released from the breakdown of glucose. This is called oxidative phosphorylation.

myelination   This is where certain neuroglia surround neuron processes called axons and form a fatty sheath which insulates it and speeds up nerve impulses. In children this process takes many years to complete and thus control of movement, for example, matures with age.

osmolality   The number of osmoles per kilogram of solvent. An osmole is a solution's ability to induce osmosis, thus it is a measurement of osmotic pressure.

parasympathetic reflexes   These nervous stimuli are initiated by the hypothalamus and result in effects of relaxation, food processing and energy absorption. The effects are usually brief and are restricted to specific organs and sites.

phagocytes   Leucocytes, usually neutrophils and monocytes. They engulf and destroy antigen–antibody complexes, bacteria, protozoa, dead cells and foreign matter.

stratum germinativum   At the epiphyseal growth plate, cartilage cells known as chondrocytes are arranged in columns extending from the epiphysis towards the shaft. The outer zone furthest from the shaft is where chondrocytes are more actively dividing. This is called the stratum germinativum.

stratum spinosum   This layer of developing bone takes its name from the process of ossification where chondrocytes hypertrophy and the lacunae around them expand to form irregular cavities in the matrix called spicules.

transient bradicardia   A short period of slow heartbeat often brought about by stimulation of the vagus nerve in the neck during intubation or passing a naso-gastric tube.

Bibliography

Chapter 1 Child physical needs

Adcock, M. (1998) 'Assessment', in K. Wilson and A. James (eds) *The Child Protection Handbook*, London: Bailliere Tindall.

American Academy of Pediatrics (1987) Committee on Sports Medicine and Committee on School Health, 'Physical fitness and the schools', *Pediatrics*, 80, 449–50.

Bee, H. (1997) *The Developing Child*, 8th edn, New York: Longman.

Berger, A. (1998) 'Human Genome Project to complete ahead of schedule', *British Medical Journal*, 317 (7162) 834.

Brown, L. and Pollitt, E. (1996) 'Malnutrition, poverty and intellectual development', *Scientific American*, February, 26–31.

Browne, K. (1998) 'Child abuse: defining, understanding and intervening', in K. Wilson and A. James (eds) *The Child Protection Handbook*, London: Bailliere Tindall.

Carter, B. and Dearmum, A. (eds) (1995) *Child Health Care Nursing*, London: Blackwell Science.

Chan, J. (1995) 'Dietary beliefs of Chinese patients', *Nursing Standard*, 9 (27) 30–4.

Department of Health (1991) *Working Together under the Children Act 1989: A Guide for Arrangements for Inter-agency Co-operation for the Protection of Children from Abuse*, London: HMSO.

——(1995) 'Infant formula and follow-on formula regulations', S1 no. 77, London: HMSO.

Fahlberg, V. (1991) *A Child's Journey Through Placement*, London: Perspective Press.

Fatchett, A. (ed.) (1995) *Childhood to Adolescence: Caring for Health*, London: Bailliere Tindall.

Gross, R. (1996) *Psychology*, 3rd edn, London: Arnold.

Hall, C. (1997) 'Children piling on the pounds … and inches', *Daily Telegraph*, 12 March, 5.

——(1999) *Daily Telegraph*, 14 January, 7.

Hall, M. B. (1996) *Health for All Children*, 3rd edn, Oxford: Oxford University Press.

Harris, R. (1998) 'Child protection, child care and child welfare', in K. Wilson and A. James (eds) *The Child Protection Handbook*, London: Bailliere Tindall.

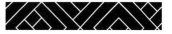

Heffernan, A. E. and O'Sullivan, A. (1998) 'Pediatric sun exposure', *The Nurse Practitioner*, 23 (7) 67–86.

Jones, D. P. H. (1991) 'The effectiveness of intervention', in M. Adcock, R. White and L. Hollows (eds) *Significant Harm: Its Outcome and Management*, Croydon: Significant Publications.

McGrath, S. A. and Gibney, M. J. (1994) 'The effects of altered frequency of eating on plasme lipids in free living healthy males on normal self-selected diets', *European Journal of Clinical Nutrition*, 48 (6) 402–7.

McQuaid, L., Huband, S. and Parker, E. (eds) (1996) *Children's Nursing*, London: Churchill Livingstone.

Moules, T. and Ramsey, J. (1998) *Children's Nursing*, Cheltenham: Stanley Thornes.

National Dairy Council (1995) 'Nutrition and teenagers: fact file 5', National Dairy Council, 5–7 John Princes Street, London W1M OAP.

Rejtman, R. (1998) 'Protecting children from disease: the debate about the MMR Vaccine', *Childright*, 146, 2–3.

Rudolf, M. and Leucene, M. (1999) *Paediatrics and Child Health*, London: Blackwell Science.

Thompson, J. (ed.) (1998) *Nutritional Requirements of Infants and Young Children*, London: Blackwell Science.

Twinn, S., Roberts, B. and Andrews, S. (1998) *Community Health Care Nursing*, Oxford: Butterworth.

Vines, G. (1997) 'Eating for two', *New Scientist*, August, 4.

White, A., Freeth, S. and O'Brian, M. (1992) *Infant Feeding OPCS Survey*, London: HMSO.

Wilsdon, J. (1993) 'The child with cerebral palsy', in A. Turner (ed.) *Occupational Therapy and Physical dysfunction*, 3rd edn, London: Churchill Livingstone.

Wilson, K. and James, A. (eds) (1998) *The Child Protection Handbook*, London: Bailliere Tindall.

Wong, D. (1996) *Clinical Manual of Pediatric Nursing*, 4th edn, St Louis MO: Mosby

——(1999) *Nursing Care of Infants and Children*, St Louis MO: Mosby.

Woodroffe, C., Glickman, M., Barker, M. and Power, C. (1993) *Children, Teenagers and Health*, Oxford: Oxford University Press.

Chapter 2   The skeletal system

Bailey, D. A. and Martin, A. D. (1994) 'Physical activity and skeletal health in adolescents', *Pediatric Exercise Science*, 6, 330–47.

Buckler J. M. H. (1994) *Growth Disorders in Children*, London: BMJ Publications.

Child Growth Foundation booklets (1994) *Growth and Growth Disorders*, Croydon: Serono Labs. *Growth Assessment in the Community*, Croydon: Pharmacia and Upjohn.

Gallo, A. M. (1996) 'Building strong bones in childhood and adolescence: reducing the risk of fractures in later life', *Pediatric Nursing*, 22 (5) 369–74.

Godderidge, C. (1995) *Pediatric Imaging*, USA: Saunders Co.

Kahn, S. A., Pace, J. E. and Cox, M. (1994) 'Osteoporosis and genetic influence: a three generation study', *Postgraduate Medical Journal*, 70 (829) 798–800.

Mathew, M. O., Ramamohan, N. and Bennet, C. (1998) 'The importance of bruising associated with paediatric fractures: a prospective observational study', *British Medical Journal*, 317, 1117–18.

Morris, F. L., Naughton, G. A., Gibbs, J. L., Carlson, J. S. and Waik, J. B. (1997) 'Prospective ten month exercise intervention in premenarcheal girls', *Journal of Bone Mineral Research*, 12, 1453–62.

Pellegrini, A. D. and Smith, P. K. (1998) 'Physical activity play: the nature and function of a neglected aspect of play', *Child Development*, 69 (3) 577–98.

Sinclair, D. (1991) *Human Growth after Birth*, 5th edn, Oxford: Oxford Medical Publications.

Tanner, J. M. (1989) *Foetus into Man*, 2nd edn, Ware: Castlemead.

Thibodeau, M. and Patton, B. (1999) *Anatomy and Physiology*, 4th edn, London: Mosby.

Voss, L. D., Mulligan, J. and Betts, P. R. (1998) 'Short stature at school entry: an index of social deprivation? Wessex Growth Study', *Child Care, Health and Development*, 24 (2) 145–56.

Chapter 3   The nervous system

Anderson, E. S., Peterson, S. A. and Wailoo, M. P. (1995) 'Factors influencing the body temperature of 3–4 months old infants at home during the day', *Archives of Disease in Childhood*, 65, 1308–10.

Atkinson, E., Vetere, A. and Grayson, K. (1995) 'Sleep disruption in young children: the influence of temperament on the sleep patterns of pre-school children', *Child Care, Health and Development*, 21 (4) 233–46.

Bee, H. (1992) *The Developing Child*, 6th edn, New York: HarperCollins.

Berne, R. M. and Levy, M. N. (1996) *Principles of Physiology*, 2nd edn, St Louis MO: Mosby.

Bliss-Holtz, J. (1993) 'Determination of thermoregulatory state in full term infants', *Nursing Research*, 42 (4) 204–7.

Campbell, S. and Glasper, E. (eds) (1995) *Children's Nursing*, London: Mosby.

Carlson, N. (1998) *Physiology of Behaviour*, 5th edn, Boston MA: Allyn and Bacon.

Edwards, S. (1998) 'High temperature', *Professional Nurse*, 13 (8) 521–6.

Goodale, M. A. (1994) 'Active minds, sleeping bodies', *The Lancet*, 344 (8929) 1036–7.

Harrison, M. (1998) 'Childhood fever: is practice scientific?', *Journal of Child Health Care*, 2 (3) 112–17.

Hinchliff, S. and Montague, S. (eds) (1998) *Physiology for Nursing Practice*, 2nd edn, London: Bailliere Tindall.

Hodgson, L. A. (1991) 'Why do we need sleep? Relating theory to nursing practice', *Journal of Advanced Nursing*, 16, 1503–10.

Kerr, S., Jowlett, S. and Smith, L. (1966) 'Preventing sleep problems in infants: a randomised controlled trial', *Journal of Advanced Nursing*, 24 (5) 938–42.

Krueger, J., Fang, J., Hanson, M., Zhang, J. and Obal, F. (1998) 'The humoral regulation of sleep', *News Physiology Science* 13, 189–94.

McQuaid, L., Hubard, S. and Parker, E. (eds) (1996) *Children's Nursing*, London: Churchill Livingstone.

Malina, R. and Bouchard, C. (1991) *Growth, Maturation, and Physical Activity*, Champaign IL: Human Kinetics Books.

Matsumura, G. and England, M. (1992) *Embryology Colouring Book*, London: Wolfe.

Mera, S. (1997) *Understanding Disease*, Cheltenham: Stanley Thornes.

Mindell, J., Moline, M., Zendell, S., Brown, L. and Fry, J. (1994) 'Pediatricians and sleep disorders: training and practice', *Pediatrics*, 94 (2) 194–200.

Nowak, T. and Handford, A. (1994) *Essentials of Pathophysiology*, Dubuque IA: Wm Brown.

O'Toole, S. (1998) 'Temperature measurement devices', *Professional Nurse*, 13 (11) 779–86.
Sinclair, D. (1991) *Human Growth after Birth*, 5th edn, Oxford: Oxford Medical Publications.
Tanner, J. M. (1989) *Foetus into Man*, 2nd edn, Ware: Castlemead Publications.
Watson, R. (1998) 'Controlling body temperature in adults', *Nursing Standard*, 12 (20) 49–53.
Watson, S. (1998) 'Using massage in the care of children', *Paediatric Nursing*, 10 (10) 27–9.
Wong, D. (1996) *Clinical Manual of Pediatric Nursing*, 4th edn, St Louis MO: Mosby.
——(1999) *Nursing Care of Infants and Children*, St Louis MO: Mosby.
Yarcheski, A. and Mahon, N. (1994) 'A study of sleep during adolescence', *Journal of Pediatric Nursing*, 9 (6) 357–66.

Chapter 4 The cardiovascular system

Armstrong, N. and Welsman, J. (1997) 'Children in sport and exercise', 1, 2, 3, *The British Journal of Physical Education*, spring, summer, winter, 30–2, 30–2, 33–4.
Gonzalez-Alonso, J. (1998) 'Separate and combined influences of dehydration and hypothermia on cardiovascular responses to exercise', *International Journal of Sports Medicine*, 19, S111–14.
Grossman, D. (1991) 'Circadian rhythms in blood pressure in school age children of normotensive and hypertensive parents', *Nursing Research*, 40 (1) 28–33.
Hazinski, M. (1992) *Nursing Care of the Critically Ill Child*, St Louis MO: Mosby.
Kelnar, C., Harvey, D. and Simpson, C. (1993) *The Sick Newborn*, London: Baillière Tindall.
Larsen, W. (1993) *Human Embryology*, Edinburgh: Churchill Livingstone.
Lissaeur, T. and Clayden, G. (1997) *Illustrated Paediatrics*, London: Mosby.
Marieb, E. (1997) *Anatomy and Physiology for Nurses*, California: Ben Cummings.
Rowland, T., Goff, D., Popowski, B., DeLuca, P. and Ferrone, L. (1998) 'Cardiac responses to exercise in child distance runners', *International Journal of Sports Medicine*, 19, 385–90.
Shuttleworth, A. (1996) 'Coronary heart disease', *Professional Nurse*, 11 (6) 386–90.
Staub, N. (1996) 'Part V Respiratory system', in R. M. Berne and M. N. Levy (eds) *Principles of Physiology*, 2nd edn, St Louis MO: Mosby.
Wong, D. (1995) *Clinical Manual of Pediatric Nursing*, 4th edn, St Louis MO: Mosby.

Chapter 5 The respiratory system

Armstrong, N. and Welsman, J. (1997a) 'Children in sport and exercise 1: bioenergetics and anaerobic exercise', *The British Journal of Physical Education*, spring, 30–2.
——(1997b) 'Children in sport and exercise 2', *The British Journal of Physical Education*, summer, 30–2.
——(1997c) 'Children in sport and exercise 3: aerobic exercise', *The British Journal of Physical Education*, winter, 33–4.

Armstrong, N., McManus, A. and Welsman, J. (1994) 'Children's aerobic fitness: children in sport and exercise', *The British Journal of Physical Education*, summer, 9–11.

British Medical Journal (1996) *Advanced Paediatric Life Support: The Practical Support*, London: BMJ.

Gregson, R., Kelly, P. and Warner, J. (1993) 'Education for control: management principles and inhaler techniques for childhood asthma', *Child Health*, June/July, 10–16.

Hazinski, M. (1992) *Nursing Care of the Critically Ill Child*, St Louis MO: Mosby.

Hlastala, M. and Berger, A. (1996) *Physiology of Respiration*, Oxford: Oxford University Press.

Kelnar, C., Harvey, D. and Simpson, C. (1993) *The Sick Newborn*, London: Bailliere Tindall.

Larsen, W. (1993) *Human Embryology*, Edinburgh: Churchill Livingstone.

Merenstein, G. B. and Gardner, S. L. (1998) *Handbook of Neonatal Intensive Care*, 4th edn, London: Mosby.

Moules, T. and Ramsey, J. (1998) *Children's Nursing*, Cheltenham: Stanley Thornes.

Rowland, T. W. (1996) *Developmental Exercise Physiology*, Champaign IL: Human Kinetics.

Strachan, D., Jarvis, M. and Feyerabend, B. (1989) 'Passive smoking, salivarycotinine concentration and middle ear effusion in 7 year old children', *British Medical Journal*, 298, 1549–52.

Wibberley, C. (1998) 'Young people's drug use: facts and feelings', *Journal of Child Health Care*, 2 (3) 138–42.

Williams, C. and Asquith, J. (eds) (2000) *Paediatric Intensive Care Nursing*, Edinburgh: Churchill Livingstone.

Wong, D. (1996) *Clinical Manual of Pediatric Nursing*, 4th edn, St Louis MO: Mosby.

Chapter 6   The renal system

Bath, R. and Morton, R. (1996) 'Nocturnal enuresis and the use of desmopressin: is it helpful?', *Child Care, Health and Development*, 22 (2) 73–84.

Bridle, R. (1994) 'Drink problem', *Nursing Times*, 90 (29) 46–7.

Burke, N. (1995) 'Alternative methods for newborn urine sample collection', *Pediatric Nursing*, 21 (6) 546.

Colborn, D. (1994) *The Promotion of Continence in Adult Nursing*, London: Chapman and Hall.

Davenport, M. (1996) 'Paediatric fluid balance', *Care of the Critically Ill*, 12 (1) 26–31.

Goin, R. (1998) 'Nocurnal enuresis in children', *Child Care, Health and Development*, 24 (4) 277–88.

Halliday, H., McClure, G. and Reid, M. (1989) *Handbook of Neonatal Intensive Care*, 3rd edn, London: Bailliere Tindall.

Larsen, W. (1993) *Human Embryology*, Edinburgh: Churchill Livingstone.

Metheny, N. (1992) *Fluid and Electrolyte Balance*, 2nd edn, New York: Lippincott Co.

Moules, T. and Ramsay, J. (1998) *Children's Nursing*, Cheltenham: Stanley Thornes.

Rogers, J. (1998) 'Nocturnal enuresis should not be ignored', *Nursing Standard*, 13 (9) 35–8.

Sinclair, D. (1991) *Human Growth after Birth*, 5th edn, Oxford: Oxford Medical Publications.

Turner, T., Douglas, J. and Cockburn, F. (1991) *Care of the Newly Born Infant*, 8th edn, Edinburgh: Churchill Livingstone.
Wong, D. (1997) *Essentials of Pediatric Nursing*, 5th edn, St Louis MO: Mosby.

Chapter 7   The digestive system

Anderson, J. (1998) 'Nappy rash: its causes, prevention and treatment', *Journal of Child Care Health*, 1 (3) 126–31.
Campbell, S. and Glasper, E. (eds) (1995) *Whaley and Wong's Children's Nursing*, London: Mosby.
Department of Health (1991) *Dietary Reference Values for Food, Energy and Nutrients for the United Kingdom: Report on Health and Social Subject No. 41*, London: HMSO.
——(1994) *Weaning and the Weaning Diet*, London: HMSO.
Gilbert, P. (1998) 'Common feeding problems in babies and children: 2', *Professional Care of Mother and Child*, 8 (3) 63–6.
Kerrigan, P. (1996) 'Management of diarrhoea by the primary health team', *Professional Care of the Mother and Child*, 2 (2) 37–8.
Lissauer, T. and Clayden, G. (1997) *Illustrated Textbook of Paediatrics*, London: Mosby.
McCance, K. and Heuther, S. (1998) *Pathophysiology: The Biological Basis for Disease in Adults and Children*, St Louis MO: Mosby.
MacKeith, R. and Wood, C. (1971) *Infant Feeding*, 4th edn, London: J. and A. Churchill.
Mascarenhas, M. R., Zemel, B. and Stallings, V. (1998) 'Nutritional assessment in pediatrics', *Nutrition*, 14, 105–15.
Moules, T. and Ramsay, J. (1998) *Children's Nursing*, Cheltenham: Stanley Thornes.
National Dairy Council (1995) 'Fact file 2: nutrition of infants and pre-school children', and 'Fact file 5: nutrition and teenagers', National Dairy Council, 5–7 John Princes Street, London W1M OAP.
Wong, D. (1996) *Clinical Manual of Pediatric Nursing*, 4th edn, St Louis MO: Mosby.

Chapter 8   The reproductive system

Berne, R. M. and Levy, M. N. (1996) *Principles of Physiology*, St Louis MO: Mosby.
Carlson, N. (1998) *Physiology of Behaviour*, 5th edn, Boston MA: Allyn and Bacon.
Chehab, F., Mounzih, K., Lu, R. and Lim, M. (1997) 'Early onset of reproductive function in normal female mice treated with leptin', *Science*, 275 (5296) 3 January, 88–90.
Chrousos, G., Torpy, D. and Gold, P. (1998) 'Interactions between the hypothalamic–pituitary–adrenal axis and the female reproductive system: clinical implications', *Annals of Internal Medicine*, 129 (3) 229–40.
Coleman, J. and Hendry, L. (1995) *The Nature of Adolescence*, London: Routledge.
Dudley, K. (1995) 'Determinedly male', *Biological Sciences Review*, January, 28–31.

Irwin, R. (1997) 'Sexual health promotion and nursing', *Journal of Advanced Nursing*, 25, (1) 170–7.

Katch, F. and McArdle, W. (1993) *Introduction to Nutrition, Exercise and Health*, 4th edn, USA: Williams and Wilkins.

Moules, T. and Ramsay, J. (1998) *Children's Nursing*, Cheltenham: Stanley Thornes.

Roberts, A. (1996) 'Glands, gender and sexuality', *Nursing Times*, 92 (7) 38–9.

Roberts, I., and Power, C. (1996) 'Does the decline in child injury mortality vary by social class?', *British Medical Journal*, 313, 784–6.

Sinclair, D. (1991) *Human Growth After Birth*, 5th edn, Oxford: Oxford Medical Publications.

Thompson, S. (1986) *Going All the Way: Teenager Girls' Tales of Sex, Romance and Pregnancy*, New York: Hill and Wang.

Wells, C. (1991) *Women, Sport and Performance*, 2nd edn, Champaign IL: Human Kinetics.

Williams, R. and Wallace, A. (1989) *Biological Effects of Physical Activity*, Champaign IL: Human Kinetics Books.

Vines, G. (1993) 'Why males live fast and die young', *New Scientist*, December, 18.

Woodroffe, C., Glickman, M., Barker, M. and Power, C. (1993) *Children, Teenagers and Health*, Oxford: Oxford University Press.

Chapter 9   The immune system

Aaby, P., Samb, B. and Simondon, F. (1995) 'Non specific beneficial effect of measles immunisation: analysis of mortality studies from developing countries', *British Medical Journal*, 311, 481–5.

Arnold, L. (ed.) (1985) *Childhood Stress*, New York: Wiley.

Campbell, J. (1992) 'A shock to the system', *Practice Nurse*, April.

——(1994) 'Making sense of immunity and immunisation', *Nursing Times*, 90 (31) 32–4.

Department of Health (1996) *Immunisation Against Infectious Disease: Edward Jenner Bicentenary Edition*, London: HMSO.

Dyson, S. (1995) 'Whooping cough vaccination: historical, social and political controversies', *Journal of Clinical Nursing*, 4, 125–31.

Frydenberg, E. (1997) *Adolescent Coping*, London: Routledge.

Groër, M. W. and Shekleton, M. E. (1989) *Pathophysiology*, London: Mosby.

Katz, S. (1997) 'Future vaccines and a global perspective', *The Lancet*, 350 (9093) 1767–70.

McCance, K. and Heuther, S. (1998) *Pathophysiology*, 3rd edn, St Louis MO: Mosby.

Matsumura, G. and England, M. (1992) *Embryology Colouring Book*, London: Wolfe.

Moules, T. and Ramsay, J. (1998) *Children's Nursing*, Cheltenham: Stanley Thornes.

Nowak, T. and Handford, A. (1994) *Essentials of Pathophysiology*, Dubuque IA: Wm Brown.

Rejtman, R. (1998) 'Protecting children from disease: the debate about the MMR Vaccine', *Childright*, 146, 2–3.

Riley, D., Mughal, M. and Roland, J. (1991) 'Immunisation state of young children admitted to hospital and effectiveness of a ward-based opportunistic immunisation policy', *British Medical Journal*, 302, 31–3.

Shucksmith, J. and Hendry, L. (1998) *Health Issues and Adolescents*, London: Routledge.

Simpson (1998) 'Infection control', *Paediatric Nursing*, 10 (10) 30–3.

Streit, W. and Kincaid-Colton, C. (1995) 'The brain's immune system', *Scientific American*, November.

Weissman, I. and Cooper, M. (1993) 'How the immune system develops', *Scientific American*, September, 65–71; 38–43.

Wong, D. (1999) *Nursing Care of Infants and Children*, St Louis MO: Mosby.

Chapter 10   Coordinating the system

Backe, B. and Nakling, J. (1998) 'Routine ultrasound dating has not been shown to be more accurate than the calendar method', *British Journal of Obstetrics and Gynaecology*, 105, 35.

Bagnell, P. (1995) 'Contracts for care: developing school health services', *Health Visitor*, 68 (9) 362–3.

Bee, H. (1995) *The Developing Child*, 7th edn, New York: HarperCollins.

Berne, R. M. and Levy, M. N. (1996) *Principles of Physiology*, St Louis MO: Mosby.

Brook, C. (1997) 'Growth hormone: panacea or punishment for short stature?', *British Medical Journal*, 315, 692–3.

Bysshe, J. (1994) 'Diagnosis and treatment of deaf babies and children', *Professional Care of Mother and Child*, August/September, 180–3.

Child Growth Foundation (1994) *Growth Assessment and Management of Growth Failure in General Practice*, London: Child Growth Foundation.

Chrousos, G., Torpy, D. and Gold, P. (1998) 'Interactions between the hypothalamic–pituitary–adrenal axis and the female reproductive system: clinical implications', *Annals of Internal Medicine*, 129(3) 229–40.

Gross, R. (1996) *Psychology*, 3rd edn, London: Arnold.

Hall, D. M. B. (1996) *Health for All Children*, 3rd edn, Oxford: Oxford University Press.

Hulse, T. (1995) 'Growth monitoring and the new growth charts', *Health Visitor*, 68 (10) 424–5.

Lightfoot, J. and Bines, W. (1997) 'Meeting the health needs of the school aged child', *Health Visitor*, 70 (2) 58–9.

Mussen, P. (1990) *Child Development and Personality*, New York: HarperCollins.

Must, A., Dallas, G. E. and Dietz, W. H. (1991) 'Reference data for 85th and 95th percentiles of body mass index and triceps skinfold thickness', *American Journal of Clinical Nutrition*, 53, 839.

Niinikoski, H., Viikari, J., Ronnemaa, T., Helenius, H., Jokinen, E., Lapinleimu, H. and Routi, T. (1997) 'Regulation of growth in 7–36 month old children by energy and fat intake in the prospective randomised strip baby trial', *Pediatrics*, 100 (5) 810–16.

Papalia, D. and Olds, S. (1992) *Human Development*, 5th edn, New York: McGraw-Hill.

Prentice, A. (1998) 'Body mass index standards for children', *British Medical Journal*, 317, 1401–2.

Rahi, J. and Dezateux, C. (1997) 'The future of preschool vision screening services in Britain', *British Medical Journal*, 315, 1247–8.

Robinson, R. (1998) 'Effective screening in child health', *British Medical Journal*, 316, 1–2.

Rudolf, M. C. J. and Levene, M. I. (1999) *Paediatrics and Child Health*, Oxford: Blackwell Science.

Sadler, C. (1998) 'Testing times ahead', *Health Visitor*, 71 (1) 7.

Steer, P. (1998) 'Fetal growth', *British Journal of Obstetrics and Gynaecology*, 105, 1133–5.

Watkin, P. and Jeremiah, Y. (1998) 'Hearing screening and the role of the health visitor', *Health Visitor*, 71 (2) 52–3.

Webb, E. (1998) 'Children and the inverse care law', *British Medical Journal*, 316, 1588–93.

Wheeler, T., Godfrey, K., Atkinson, C., Badger, J., Kay, R., Owens, R. and Osmond, C. (1998) 'Disproportionate fetal growth and fingerprint patterns', *British Journal of Obstetrics and Gynaecology*, 105, 562–4.

Wong, D. (1996) *Clinical Manual of Pediatric Nursing*, St Louis MO: Mosby.

——(1999) *Essentials of Pediatric Nursing*, St Louis MO: Mosby.

Index

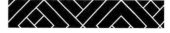